362.43
MOR

...omen's Press Ltd
...Great ...on Street, London EC1V 0DX

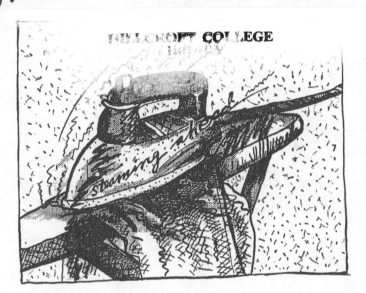

In 1984 after two conferences organised by the Spinal Injuries Association, a group of spinal cord injured women came together for the purpose of compiling this book. The editorial group comprises:

Lesley Broomhead
Lydia Cooke
Judy Crosby
Maggie Davis
Ann Duncan
Enid King
Diana Levett
Jenny Morris
Joanna Owen
Diane Pargetter
Patricia Pay
Sue Sharp
Anne Spooner
Rosalie Wilkins
Lucina Willan
Margaret Williams

Jenny Morris, editor

Able Lives

Women's Experience of Paralysis

Illustrated by Angela Martin

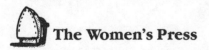 The Women's Press

First published by The Women's Press Limited 1989
A member of the Namara Group
34, Great Sutton Street, London EC1V 0DX

British Library Cataloguing in Publication Data
available

Typeset by Boldface Typesetters, London EC1
Printed and bound in Great Britain by Hazell, Watson
and Viney Ltd, Aylesbury, Bucks.

Tomorrow I Am Going To Re-write The English Language

Tomorrow I am going to re-write the English Language.
I will discard all those striving ambulist metaphors
Of power and success
And construct new images to describe my strength.
My new, different strength.

Then I won't have to feel dependent
Because I can't Stand On My Own Two Feet
And I will refuse to feel a failure
Because I didn't Stay One Step Ahead.
I won't feel inadequate
When I don't Stand Up For Myself
Or illogical because I cannot
Just Take It One Step at a Time.

I will make them understand that it is a very male way
To describe the world
All this Walking Tall
And Making Great Strides.

Yes, tomorrow I am going to re-write the English Language,
Creating the world in my own image.
Mine will be a gentler, more womanly way
To describe my progress.
I will wheel, cover and encircle

Somehow I will learn to say it all.

Lois Keith

Contents

Acknowledgements

The Editorial Group would like to pay tribute to the 205 women on whose returned questionnaires this book is based. For many it was a painful experience to write of their injury and its aftermath. Our common concern, however, was to share such personal experiences in the hope that the isolation of disability would be diminished.

We would also like to thank Frances Hasler, the Spinal Injury Association's Welfare Officer, and Mandy Hooper who succeeded Frances. They provided all the administrative support that was needed and their warm enthusiasm was much appreciated.

Finally, this book was made possible through the existence of the Spinal Injuries Association, the organisation run by spinal cord injured people on behalf of spinal cord injured people and their families and friends. The SIA provided the financial and administrative support for the women's conferences at which this book originated and then made it financially and practically possible to send out the questionnaires, for them to be analysed and for many meetings of the 16-strong Editorial Group to be held. We hope the book is a fitting testimony to the value of collective action by disabled people.

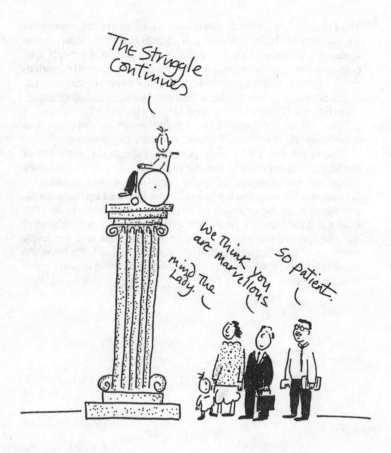

Introduction

This book is about a group of people from many different backgrounds, in a variety of circumstances, and with a whole range of feelings and politics. We have two things in common, however. We are all women and we have all experienced a spinal cord injury resulting in varying degrees of paralysis. We therefore share a common position in our relationship to other people and to society in general. We are restricted not only by the physical handicap itself but by the way we are set apart from other people, the way our concerns are ignored and the stereotypes applied to us.

Part of our oppression is caused by our isolation from one another. This is one of the reasons for this book: to share our experiences with each other. Another reason is to make public our concerns and difficulties, and to express our anger at the way in which non-disabled people handicap us, both by their attitudes and their organisation of the physical environment.

In 1984, the Spinal Injuries Association (a self-help organisation run by spinal cord injured people) held two national Women's Conferences, where, in many cases for the first time, women shared their experiences of disability. The idea for this book came out of those conferences. We felt there was a need for us to publish our experiences, as one woman said at the time, 'I would have given a great deal to have been able to read about how other women felt instead of having to lock up my unanswered questions inside myself.' We also felt there was a need to make disability more familiar to the general public.

After the conferences, a group of 16 spinal cord injured women came together to devise a questionnaire which was then sent out to all women members of the Spinal Injuries Association. This book is based on the answers to the questions contained in the questionnaires which were returned.

What is spinal cord injury?

Spinal cord injury can be at different levels and cause varying degrees of paralysis. Some of us can walk with crutches and calipers; some are wheelchair users but with a range of abilities, from having full use of our hands and arms to very little use of either. Paralysis also affects the bladder and bowels, making incontinence a major part of disability. There are many causes of spinal cord injury, ranging from sudden damage to the cord caused by a car accident to gradual damage caused by a tumour.

Spinal cord injured people tend to use a certain amount of jargon relating to their condition. The spinal column protecting the spinal cord is divided into four sections of vertebrae: cervical (neck), thoracic (trunk) and lumbar and sacral (at the base of your spine). The level of injury to the spinal cord is referred to by the level of vertebra at which it occurs, thus 'C5' means injury at the level of the fifth cervical vertebra. We also sometimes talk about 'incomplete' and 'complete'. This simply means whether the damage to the cord was total, with complete loss of feeling and function below that level, or whether partial damage resulted in incomplete feeling and/or function.

Tetraplegia (or quadraplegia, which is the American term) means that the lesion (damage) to the spinal cord was at the cervical level and that the upper part of the body, including the arms and hands, as well as the lower part of the body, is paralysed. What function there is in a person's hands and arms, and whether or not there is any feeling, will depend both on the level of injury to the neck and if the lesion was complete or incomplete. Paraplegia arises from damage to the spinal cord at thoracic or lumbar level, involving paralysis

Spine, Spinal Cord and Nerve Supply

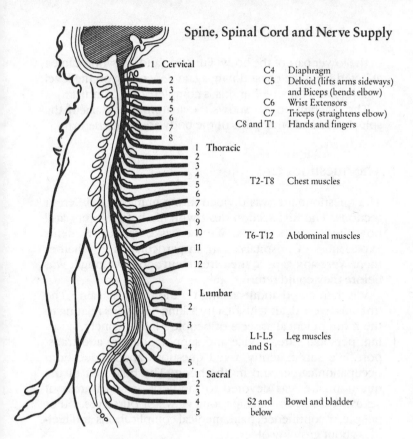

1 Cervical
2
3
4
5
6
7
8

C4	Diaphragm
C5	Deltoid (lifts arms sideways) and Biceps (bends elbow)
C6	Wrist Extensors
C7	Triceps (straightens elbow)
C8 and T1	Hands and fingers

1 Thoracic
2
3
4
5
6
7
8
9
10
11
12

T2-T8	Chest muscles
T6-T12	Abdominal muscles

1 Lumbar
2
3
4
5

L1-L5 and S1	Leg muscles

1 Sacral
2
3
4
5

S2 and below	Bowel and bladder

The diagram illustrates the spinal column divided into its four groups of vertebrae, cervical, thoracic, lumbar and sacral. Also indicated are the groups of muscles in the body which are affected by damage to the spinal cord at the different levels of vertebrae.

The spinal cord is made up of thousands of nerve fibres linking the brain with the various parts of the body. It is encased within the vertebrae which make up the spine. If this vital communication between the brain and the rest of the body is broken, messages about feeling and movement cannot get through.

Whatever level at which damage to the spinal cord occurs, it is not just the area of the body related to that part of the spinal cord which is affected but all the body below that level as well. Thus, an injury at the level of the eighth cervical vertebra (C8) will affect not only the hands and fingers but also the chest, abdomen, legs, and bladder and bowels. The extent of injury to the spinal cord (how badly it is crushed) will determine the extent of paralysis, that is, whether or not there is complete loss of feeling and movement below a particular level.

Adapted from
'So You're Paralysed . . .'
© Liz McQuiston

of the lower part of the body. Function and sensation can be affected from the chest down, again depending on the level of injury and on whether this is complete or incomplete.

The diagram on p.3 shows the anatomical details of the spinal cord and what parts of the body are affected.

The questionnaire

The questionnaire was divided into a number of different sections. The first section dealt with life before injury and how the injury occurred. We then asked about women's experiences of hospitalisation, in particular as to whether there were any gaps in their treatment and how long it was before they could return home.

We then asked about 'taking up the threads again'. The 'threads' were dealt with first by asking questions relating to the more practical aspects of people's lives, namely, housing, personal care, advice and support, money and transport. We subsequently asked questions about education/ occupation/career and motherhood. The final part of the questionnaire was devoted to the very personal areas of sexuality and relationships, our views of ourselves, other people, incontinence, pain, medical complications and feelings about growing older.

How we wrote this book

A group of 16 women came together after the 1984 Women's Conferences to devise the questionnaire, analyse the results and write the book. As the completed questionnaires were returned, each member of the editorial group took a section of each questionnaire to analyse, and we began the slow process of circulating each one around the group. Every member of the editorial group wrote an initial draft chapter using quotes from the questionnaires. One member (Jenny Morris) then took on the task of pulling all the chapters together into a common format and style.

The book is divided into areas of all our lives rather than focusing on the whole life experience of a few women. We felt that this format would be the one most useful to other disabled women as it would help them dip into parts of the book that were of most interest to them at any one particular stage of their lives. We also wanted to avoid presenting an 'elite' of disabled women who were coping wonderfully – because the majority of us do not feel like that about ourselves. Such books only make us feel inadequate.

This book differs from other books about and by disabled people in that it deals with the very nitty gritty and personal details of living with disability, issues of which the non-disabled world is mainly ignorant because they are not generally talked about. Books which specify how 'wonderful' disabled people are don't in fact deal with the sometimes humiliating consequences of bladder and bowel incontinence, or how someone might feel about not being able to have an orgasm ever again. Yet such issues are central to the way we feel about ourselves and our relationships with other people.

The questionnaires were known to those of us who analysed them only by their numbers. We have given each number a fictional name which has been used for extracts from that questionnaire which appear throughout the book. The information therefore remains anonymous, but brief biographical details are given for each 'name' at the back of the book.

For a postal questionnaire involving open-ended questions, the response rate was quite good – 205 (29 per cent) of the 700 questionnaires were answered and returned. We would like to think that the book speaks, to some extent, for the many women who did not reply – and, of course, for those who are not even members of the Spinal Injuries Association. Amongst those who replied, 38 (almost one in five) were over 60; another 89 (two in five) were aged between 40 and 59, 65 (one-third) were 25–39 and the rest (13 women) were aged 16–24. There was also a fairly good spread in terms of both level of paralysis, cause and length of time paralysed.

Even within a 'minority group' of disabled women there are further minorities. Those of us who are tetraplegic, or older, or whose injury was gradual rather than the result of an accident, or those who are able to walk with crutches, often feel isolated by the stereotypical young, fit, independent wheelchair user. Our questionnaire was returned by women who fit all these descriptions, and their experiences are fully represented in this book.

As the questionnaire was not part of a piece of social science research but was set up to enable women to write about their experiences and feelings, we were not able to classify according to class or ethnic origin. We could not therefore assess whether working class or black women were fully represented numerically, although we did make a special effort to try to increase the response rate amongst ethnic minority women members of the SIA.

The representation of lesbians in the book was also problematic as although a number of the questions were specifically related to sexuality and relationships only a few women actually identified themselves as lesbian. We tried to rectify this by appealing through the SIA Newsletter for lesbian spinal cord injured women to fill in the questionnaire and by contacting GEMMA (an organisation for disabled and able-bodied lesbians). Unfortunately, however, we had no further response. We feel sure that a number of women who did fill in the questionnaire were lesbians but did not wish to write about this.

The editorial group have used the questionnaires that *have* been returned by working class, black and ethnic minority women, and lesbians to give voices to such women. We certainly do not want to collude in the way in which such women are usually treated – as invisible – for becoming invisible is, of course, exactly what happens to women with disabilities. We would therefore ask you, the reader, not to assume that the women you are reading about are necessarily white, middle class and heterosexual; they may well not be.

Our aim has been to write a book about women's lives. It is a book of voices that are too often silenced. It is not intended to be a handbook (although we have included a brief list of resources at the back), or to be a treatise on 'what should be done'. We want to share our experiences, to help newly disabled women and to help dispel the ignorance and misunderstandings about disability amongst both the general public and the health and social service 'experts'.

The book is about the reality of our lives and there is pain as well as joy. The concern of the editorial group was not to impose a particular perspective on any of the women who filled in our questionnaires but to enable publication of their writings about the reality of their lives. The message is neither how awful life is for a disabled woman, nor how wonderful we all are. If we have a message it is anger at how our concerns as spinally injured women are isolated within each individual's private world and so very rarely made part of the public world. When we 'appear' as a public issue it is usually in the way the non-disabled world defines us and our concerns, and not in the way we would wish to appear ourselves.

This book is a small attempt to bring us out into the open and to make us less invisible in the eyes of non-disabled people. Primarily, however, we hope that it will speak to disabled women and that by sharing our experiences we will in some way help to counteract the isolation of disability.

1.

Injury and Loss

Spinal cord injury is not only medically traumatic; it affects a person most profoundly, and shatters a way of life. It divides an individual's history into two – before and after the event (or sometimes series of events) and marks the transition to disability. Many of us stress our abilities rather than what we are not able to do, but we usually find it impossible to escape from the social definition given to us by non-disabled people as 'unable'. Overnight we become part of a marginalised group: outsiders, objects of fear, pity, or patronising wonder at how well we 'manage'.

In fact, the ways of seeing and treatment of those of us who were not born disabled, but who suddenly pass over the line from 'normal' to 'abnormal', blatantly exposes the prejudice and ignorance that all disabled people encounter. An important part of our experience following spinal cord injury is the realisation that we have been plummetted over this line. Our bewilderment, grief and anger at our physical state may well be aggravated by the social experiences resulting from our sudden, enforced membership of one of the most discriminated against groups in society.

Much of the material in this book illustrates how it is other people and the physical environment which really handicap us. Essentially we remain the same people after our injury as we were before. However, the restrictions and frustrations that now form part of our lives mean that many of us look back to the time before injury with nostalgia; sometimes with intense regret for the unsuspecting people we were then – a time of irretrievable 'normality'.

How did it happen?

We asked the women taking part in this project to describe the cause of their injuries. The answers illustrate how spinal cord injury can happen to anyone, at any time, and just how dangerous life can sometimes be – not just obvious road traffic or dangerous sports accidents.

Non-traumatic injuries (that is, injury caused by illness or medical conditions) are a fairly common cause of spinal cord injury for women. Some of us who experienced non-traumatic injury tend to feel isolated, and that we have little in common with those whose paralysis was caused by an accident. In fact, 53 (one in four) who answered the questionnaire were paralysed as a result of a medical condition or illness. The single most common medical cause was a growth (tumour, abscess or cyst) which accounted for 13 injuries to the spinal cord. Eleven women were paralysed as a result of an operation. A virus, transverse myelitis, accounted for another eight women's paralysis, while an unspecified virus infection accounted for another five. Eleven women either did not know or did not specify the medical condition wich caused their paralysis.

The circumstances of becoming paralysed as a result of a medical condition can add to our anguish. For example, Bernadette, paralysed as a result of degeneration of the spinal cord from pernicious anaemia (a blood disorder) writes, 'It was quite traumatic how it happened. I just collapsed on the floor in [the] hospital and could not get up. I never walked again. After three months in this hospital, I was sent to the spinal injury unit . . . where I stayed seven months. When it happened I was 44 years old. The doctors never told me I would not be able to walk again. I was just left to work it out for myself.'

For Ruth, the attitudes of the hospital staff were more distressing than the disease itself. 'In 1951 at the age of 21, I had a tumour which crushed the spinal cord. The doctors took three years to find out what was wrong but by the time they did I was paralysed. They said I was mental and put me in a mental hospital. When I fell down they would hit me. I had to cope with the pain and the fear of falling. It was a terrible time.'

Fiona also had a spinal tumour, but it was medical intervention which actually paralysed her. A doctor herself, she writes that the tumour was first discovered in 1968 when she was 35. 'I had a biopsy and radiotherapy with good result. I was quite frail for a few months, then well. I got more unsteady in 1980–81 but was not using a stick or other aid. The tumour was reinvestigated and recurrence suspected. Urgent surgery was advised, which I resisted for three months. I was then operated on with a laser but it did not go well! There was no evidence of recurrence of the tumour and I've been a paraplegic since.'

The single most common cause of spinal cord injury is, however, road traffic accidents. Of the 90 women injured in this way, some were drivers or passengers in a car, while others were pedestrians. Many of our stories illustrate the terrible suddenness of such accidents. Elsa was on her way home from church with her husband and two small children when the whole family was ploughed into on the pavement by a speeding car. 'My daughter (aged 7) was fatally injured, dying four days later in a London hospital. My husband was very severely injured and in intensive care, but is now fit enough to work. My son (aged 4) escaped injury and was cared for by local friends. I was paralysed at T12 and had a fractured elbow with subsequent ulna nerve injury [which restricts use of the arm].'

Marion had been waiting (with her husband and 26-year-old daughter) for the AA on the hard shoulder of the M11 for two hours when another car drove into the back of their car at high speed (and in broad daylight). She was 51 years old. 'I am now paralysed at T6 complete. I was also paralysed completely down my right side from a head injury. This has affected my speech but I am regaining a little strength back in my right arm, although it will never be as strong as the left arm.'

Linda is generous in absolving anyone of any blame for her accident. Aged 33 and with a 13-year-old daughter, she was a passenger in the car which her husband was driving.

'Because the weather was bad, a petrol tanker had decided to use the B road. He wasn't in the wrong but there just wasn't room for all of us. We caught the bank and over-turned. . . . The worst moment was coming round in the inside roof of the upturned car next to the middle of the road, unable to move, with cars insisting on driving through, inches away from me.'

Falls (other than industrial injury or suicide attempts) accounted for 25 women's injuries. Rachel did not fall from any great height. 'I was 38 years old and on the last Friday in August 1981 I finished work for a month's holiday and went out with a few friends to celebrate. Later I went home and as the night was very warm I didn't feel able to sleep so I went outside to sit on a wall and look at the sea. It was a narrow wall with a drop of just over one metre to the other side. There are drainage holes in the wall and children had pushed lengths of wood into the holes. I overbalanced and landed on the wood fracturing my first lumbar vertebra.'

Wendy became a tetraplegic following a fall down a flight of stairs in her own home. She was in her 30s with teenage children. Blanche's experience also demonstrates the dangers that lurk in our homes: 'It was the end of May 1961. I was 31. Not feeling very well I tried to pull myself together by getting on with sealing the leaks in my workroom attic window. I blacked out and came to as I was going over the edge of the roof.' She is now an incomplete paraplegic, walking with sticks.

A domestic setting also proved dangerous for Libby. 'I was just 17½ when I broke my neck. It happened in the block of flats where I lived (and still live). It is a Victorian mansion block where the stairs go up round a lift shaft protected by a metal railing, which only came up to "neck" height. It was possible to look down the lift shaft to see people coming up the stairs, which is what happened on the evening of 19 August 1980. I was going out with friends that evening. Two of them had arrived but one was late, and so when she finally arrived I rushed out on to the landing and, without thinking, looked down the shaft. The lift came down and hit me on the back of the head, causing lacerations on my chin, neck and the back of my head (all leaving bad scars) and a dislocation of the C4 and C5 vertebrae. Although completely paralysed for about a month afterwards, I was very lucky and regained much muscle power. I can walk but have to use a stick; my gait is slow and uneven and I tire very easily. I have quite a lot of spasticity [involuntary muscle contractions] so my left foot, especially, tends to drag and my left hand has limited movement. Sensation is also affected but I have no numb patches.'

Three of us were paralysed as a result of suicide attempts. One of these was Alice who describes what happened when she was 24 years old. 'I had had a tape worm on returning from Kenya and the treatment made me very hypermanic. I was given electric shock treatment for this . . . I left the hospital with no after-care and gave myself my own shock treatment by jumping off a roof, but it did restore my sanity! I am paraplegic but now incomplete . . . I walk resolutely with sticks as well as using a wheelchair.'

Paralysis was just part of very traumatic events for Paula and Ranjan, both of whom were stabbed. Paula was stabbed 13 times in the back and head by her husband, while Ranjan's mother was killed in the same assault in which she was paralysed at the age of nine.

Six of us were injured at work, another six in sporting activity and 12 as a result of horse-riding accidents. Gillian, a 23-year-old teacher at the time of her injury, describes her climbing accident. 'I was rock climbing with three friends in Snowdonia. I led the climb and at about 20 feet from the summit of Tryfan the rock and I parted company. I fell from ledge to ledge, about 45 feet. To this day it isn't known how or why I fell.'

Sometimes paralysis can strike many years after an accident which damaged the spine. This was Joyce's experience. She first hurt her back when she fell off a horse in 1960. In 1968 she stuck, bent doubled up when changing a wheel on her car. She had an operation in 1971 but in 1980 was again suddenly stuck doubled up. Following a second operation she is now paralysed from the waist.

Violet has gradually become more paralysed but can trace

the cause back to the day of the Aberfan disaster when she fell down stairs at work. 'My life changed completely that day,' she wrote. After a major operation on her back, she was able to walk with two sticks and was given a desk job. 'I was medically retired in 1977 and am now in a wheelchair with acute pain. I am told it will get worse.'

Our descriptions of our lives 'before' illustrate how disability can happen to anyone. Overnight we become strange, alien, *different* as far as the able-bodied world is concerned – we stick out like a sore thumb in most public places, whereas the day before our injury we would have passed unnoticed.

An important part of the able-bodied world's inability to treat us the same as anyone else is a lack of understanding that disability can, and does, happen to anyone. Who would have thought, for example, that Mary, a 25-year-old mother of a 15-month-old child would suddenly become paralysed as the result of a car accident while on holiday in Ireland? She describes her life at the time of her accident. 'I had left teaching to have my first child in June 1977. In September 1977 I enrolled for night school studying psychology and also played volleyball with friends from my old college one evening per week. My days were spent looking after my daughter, taking her swimming and out to parks and places of interest. In October 1978 we were on holiday in Ireland when our accident happened.'

Paralysis was equally sudden for Sandra, even though it was not the result of an accident. 'I was 30 years old and married with three young children. Having had three children in four years I was very active, but social life was, of necessity, limited. Also I had had back trouble since the birth of my third child. On 5 March 1975, I had a back operation, after which I got a blood clot on the spinal cord. I became paralysed from the waist down.'

What have we lost?

Disability as a result of injury (following an accident or

illness) is primarily about loss – loss of ability, loss of the taken-for-granted life before the momentous event (or events). In fact, most of us carry on our lives in much the same way as before our injury, as this book shows, although at the time of injury it is difficult to understand how this can ever be possible. Many of us, however, are filled with regret and a sense of loss when we look back.

Norma was injured when only 16 years old, and overnight was confronted with a lifetime of disability. She writes of her life before her injury. 'It was very enjoyable. I was a typical teenager. I had left school at 15 and was employed as a copy typist in the City. I had a steady boyfriend and we had, in fact, just got engaged. I loved dancing, ice skating, swimming and window shopping (we didn't have much money or a car so this was a favourite pastime). On 29 December 1959, I had just left my sister at the station when I went to cross the main road and was hit by a lorry. The extent of permanent injury was a broken neck, C6 complete.'

Twenty-two-year-old Olivia stresses the full and active nature of her previous life. 'I was living with my boyfriend in his house. I was working full-time as a secretary and he works away from home. I was interested in hiking, hockey, motor bikes, men and alcohol. I cycled to work (14 miles round trip), went jogging and swimming. Life was conducted at high speed; work was five days when I slowed down a bit and nursed hangovers in preparation for the weekend! I was reckless, impetuous and only vaguely planned ahead. My mother furiously disapproved of my life style; my father never commented on it.'

Olivia's love of life is echoed by June who was 57 at the time of her accident. 'I was on top of the world. Life was wonderful. I had just retired from a professional situation, after working since leaving school at 14. I am happily married, have one daughter living near, and three lovely grandchildren. I had a full social life, regular nights out with colleagues, local dances and outings with grandchildren.'

However, not all of us focus on what we have lost from our lives before our injury. Frances, for example, emphasises the continuity in her life. 'I was a student doing a degree in Law and Politics. I was in the last term of my final year of the degree which was a continuous assessment course, so despite the fact I missed the last set of exams I still got my degree. I was, and still am, single. I was, and still am, a very social person. I love parties, including giving dinner parties.'

Brenda, who was 52 when she had a riding accident, also writes about continuity. She carried on running her farm, in spite of both her injury and her husband's death from cancer 14 months after her accident. She says: 'I was an active farmer's wife helping both outside with animals and normal running of the house, etc. After my husband's death I decided to continue running the farm within a partnership. My partner deals with the outside and I run the office.'

Moreover, some of us have little regret for the life which we lost. Isabel writes of her life before her suicide attempt at the age of 18. 'I did not have much of a social life but I put up a cheerful facade at times. I was asthmatic and a very closeted lesbian. In fact I had no word for my sexuality – gayness was never talked about. It was an anaesthetised sort of life, a half life, really.'

Isabel writes later on in this book of the positive things that are now happening in her life and many of us are able to do this, even when we have regrets for what we have lost. Life is by no means rosy, and some of us are in despair, but the women who have contributed to this book demonstrate that disability does not necessarily mean living a life which is of a poorer quality in all aspects. In many respects it is circumstances other than disability – whether we have suitable housing, enough money, people who love us – that determine the quality of our lives.

This is so even when our injuries were part of an event which tore our families' lives apart. Madeleine is someone whose accident resulted in such devastation: 'I was married with three small children (3, 2 and 3 months at the time of the accident) . . . We had a car crash. My husband fell asleep, tired from overwork. He was thrown out of the car and killed, I was jammed in it and became C7 incomplete (left side) and T3 complete (right side).' The effect of the accident on her daughter demonstrates how their lives were shattered – and then re-built. 'The 3-year-old started school when she was 4 and I was still in hospital. When I got home, the teacher showed me her paintings. The ones done when I was in hospital were wild splodges of black and red. When I first came home they became multi-coloured. Within a few weeks they were pale spring colours of blue, green, yellow.'

Conclusion

This chapter has introduced the reader to the trauma of spinal cord injury and also to some of the women who feature in this book. However positive our lives after injury, the crossing over into the world of disability means that our accident or illness marks a fundamental change. The next chapter looks at our experience of hospitalisation, for this is the first stage in the rest of our lives.

2.

Hospitals

This chapter is about our experience of hospitals and their associated professionals (doctors, nurses, occupational and physiotherapists, and social workers), following spinal cord injury. We have widely differing experiences and views on the quality and content of treatment and care. Some of us were recounting experiences of 30 years ago, while others had only recently become paralysed. Hospitals differ in their methods of treatment and rehabilitation and there have also been some changes over time. Our opinions of the standards of care were influenced not only by what was offered to us but also by what we brought to the situation. However, we all found that our first experiences after injury were not just straightforward medical reactions to our paralysis but more general reactions to disability and the consequences of this.

Spinal cord injury, especially if it is caused by an accident, means months in hospital. Traumatic injury usually requires eight to ten weeks spent flat on your back while the vertebrae stabilise to prevent further damage to the spinal cord. Sometimes surgery is carried out (involving grafting bone on to the damaged vertebra or the insertion of a metal plate); this enables sitting up within a few weeks rather than two to three months. The period of time spent in bed following a non-traumatic injury to the spinal cord (for example, a virus or tumour) will depend on the nature of the medical condition.

Once this initial phase is over, what the professionals call 'rehabilitation' begins. In a spinal unit this will involve fairly

intensive physiotherapy and, possibly, occupational therapy. It comes as a surprise to many newly injured paraplegics and tetraplegics that the first physical obstacle to overcome is to relearn how to balance. Before paralysis we
unconsciously use our legs and feet to balance, even when
sitting down. Now our centre of gravity has changed and we
have to learn to balance from the waist, the chest or the
shoulders, depending on the level of lesion.

Having learnt to balance, we can then start to learn all the
things which will determine what level of personal independence we will have: getting dressed, getting in and out of the
wheelchair, pushing the wheelchair, lifting it in and out of a
car. If we have lost strength in our arms and dexterity in our
fingers, we will spend time learning to make the most of
what movement we have. All this requires strength in the
muscles left to us, and therefore a lot of time is spent doing
muscle-building exercises.

During the months in hospital we become experts in preventing pressure sores, dealing with incontinence, coping
with body temperature problems and other aspects of living
with paralysis. But 'rehabilitation' is not just about physical
matters, although professionals sometimes behave as if this
were in fact the case. We are involved in adapting all aspects
of our lives. Probably the most important thing that has to
be sorted out is suitable housing, the lack of which can delay
discharge from hospital for many months. There are also
very many other practical and emotional things to cope
with, ranging from how we are going to look after our children, whether or not we can go back to work, to what is
going to happen to our sexual relationships. Hospitals and
the professionals who run them can be crucial in helping us
to confront these issues. Sadly, they usually fail us.

This chapter focuses on various aspects of our experience
of hospitalisation, highlighting the difficulties which occur.
First, three women write of the trauma and general upheaval
which sudden and long hospitalisation brings.

Helen describes her experience following the sudden
onset of paralysis due to a viral infection when she was 27
years old. She had a 13-month-old daughter and was two

months pregnant. 'I was in a general hospital initially, then moved to a spinal unit after one month. The doctors in the general hospital left me totally unaware of the gloomy prognosis and it was only when I was transferred to the spinal unit that I realised the permanency of the paralysis. During the two months I spent in the spinal unit, I could hardly grasp all the things which were going to change in our lives. I was discharged early because I was eight weeks pregnant when paralysed and when I got to 20 weeks, physio and other rehabilitation were becoming too difficult for me.'

Her baby was born brain damaged by the virus which had paralysed her and only lived five days.

Lynne became a tetraplegic in 1979 at the age of 18, following a car accident. 'Initially I was admitted to a general orthopaedic ward in the local hospital. I spent the first month there. The consultant and nursing staff were not experienced in treating spinal injury, although they were very supportive to my family and friends. I got a text book version of my injury explained to me 10 days after it had happened, which included the consultant telling me that I would never walk again – which I didn't believe because I had picked up their general lack of knowledge about what had happened and how to treat me. I was on a stryker frame [a bed which can be turned upside down to relieve pressure areas] which absolutely terrified me, and was in a lot of pain due to a broken arm which had also happened as a result of the crash. When I went to the spinal unit it suddenly hit me that I wasn't going to walk again – when I saw everyone else whizzing around in wheelchairs. I had little professional counselling on what had actually happened and how this would affect my physical state.'

Erica had had a long history of back problems, culminating in surgery in 1982. She was in her early 40s with teenage children. 'I spent over one year in a general hospital on an orthopaedic ward before being transferred to a spinal unit. Looking back it is difficult to understand why I was kept in for so long. I had continual tests and attempts at treatments and I think my unquestioning acceptance of being incarcerated was based on the feeling that whilst still in hospital there was hope that there would be a cure. Despite a very caring consultant I felt very alone and frightened after not being told any reason for the treatment or the stopping of it. I always felt that I wasn't told enough about my condition or asked how I felt. I had an overwhelming feeling of guilt towards my husband and children, knowing the difficulties of their situation. It was not until my transfer to a spinal unit that I had to face the realities and rather than live on hope I learnt and accepted my limitations. I spent three months in the spinal unit and during that time began to piece my life together positively.'

Getting the treatment we need

Women who are not admitted to spinal injury units are less likely to receive the specialist medical treatment and rehabilitation services they need. They are also less likely to come into contact with the Spinal Injuries Association. Generally, someone whose spinal cord injury is owing to an illness, tumour or abscess (that is, non-traumatic) and/or where paralysis comes on over a period of time, is less likely to be referred to a spinal unit. Women are more likely to experience this type of spinal cord injury than men, a larger proportion of whose injuries are caused by road traffic and sporting accidents.

The subject of the 'invisibility' of women who never get to a spinal unit is important, first because it is generally agreed that admission to a spinal unit is vital, not only for whatever medical or surgical treatment we may need but also to get the best chances of returning to an independent life. Secondly, it is clear from our experiences that spinal units do not address the particular needs of women, and they are unlikely to do so while women continue to be underrepresented in both spinal units as patients and in the official statistics on spinal cord injury.

Forty-five out of the total 205 women who answered the questionnaire never went to a spinal unit. From the experience of women whose paralysis was due to an accident, it seems that the chances of going to a spinal unit increased significantly after 1960 but do not appear to have continued to increase. Amongst these women who experienced traumatic injury, 29 per cent of those injured before 1959 never went to a spinal unit. After 1960 this figure dropped to 10 per cent and has remained at that level.

For women experiencing non-traumatic injury (53) the figures are too small to give an accurate picture of whether or not the chances of admission to a spinal unit have changed over the years. However, it is clear that women who are paralysed as a result of a non-traumatic injury are less likely to get into a spinal unit – 35 per cent of those experiencing immediate paralysis and 85 per cent of those who became paralysed over a period of time never went to a spinal unit.

This lack of specialist treatment can make our lives much more difficult. The inadequacies of general hospitals are demonstrated by the experience of someone such as Tessa who writes of the unsatisfactory nature of her treatment in 1979 at a well-known teaching hospital: 'I was given no practical help with how to transfer, dress, balance, get into a car, etc.' She experienced a common disadvantage of remaining in a general hospital: there was no one in a similar situation to her and therefore no one to talk to about what was happening and the treatment she was receiving. She was aged 20 at the time of the illness which paralysed her.

The gaps in the treatment given by general hospitals are also illustrated by Vicky's experience. She was in a general hospital neurological unit for a year in 1974–5 where 'the initial treatment was excellent but the rehabilitation terrible. I learned nothing about actually living with a wheelchair and was sent home for my first weekend without a cushion for my wheelchair [something which was bound to result in a pressure sore]. There was no one to talk to. I never met another fully rehabilitated paraplegic or tetraplegic.'

A lack of specialist treatment can lead to serious medical problems, the most common being pressure sores and bladder problems. Many women who spent some time in a general hospital before being transferred to a spinal unit arrived at the spinal unit with pressure sores. Marion recounted her experience of nearly six months in a general hospital in 1983. 'I felt an outsider. No one knew enough about how to treat a paralysed patient; when to lift and turn to prevent bedsores. As it was all new to me I did not know about pressure areas and I got a pressure sore.'

However, whatever our criticisms of general hospitals, we also have many criticisms of the spinal units. There are nine specialist spinal units in England and Wales, two in Scotland, one in Northern Ireland and one in Eire. While a few of us praised the excellent treatment received, more were critical of the care, rehabilitation and general support that was experienced in these centres. One particular criticism, common amongst women of all ages, was that there was little or no help in coming to terms with the emotional upheaval caused by the trauma of sudden paralysis. Some of us highlighted this as the only fault in an otherwise satisfactory rehabilitation, but for others this problem affected the whole experience of hospitalisation. The failure to address the emotional aspects of our injury was also associated with other criticisms which centred around the way in which women's concerns were ignored, the quality of care and a failure to help us plan our future. The rest of this chapter explores these criticisms under separate headings, although inevitably there is an overlap between the different concerns.

Feelings

Our most common criticism of general hospitals and spinal units was of the way the professionals seemed to ignore our feelings about the situation in which we suddenly found ourselves. Bridget, who was in a general hospital for 2½ weeks and at a spinal unit for 4½ months, remembered: 'I was appalled at the seeming callousness of the nurses and, as a feminist, I found their attitude very hard to come to terms with. There was no one in either hospital who seemed at all interested in how I felt. I twice tried to express my grief but was met with a total lack of response.'

Some of us did recognise that nurses were often working under difficult conditions of staff shortages, but many, like Libby, still did not feel that this excused 'the brisk and often callous attitude of the doctors and nurses'. The overwhelming message from women's experience of treatment and rehabilitation following spinal cord injury is that, with some exceptions, there seems to be a policy, and there is certainly a practice, of giving very little attention to the emotional aspects of treatment and rehabilitation.

This is illustrated by Shirley's remark that although 'the treatment was OK, one was not allowed to break down and cry. A stiff upper lip was called for.' And Rosemary felt that 'the staff expected you to have a smile on your face all the time'. This is one aspect of hospital treatment which seems to be as common now as it was 20 or 30 years ago.

Nora wrote of her experience in hospital following her accident. 'I had regular physiotherapy and did occupational therapy, but there was no one to discuss problems and personal feelings with, and no form of counselling to help with the present or future. It seemed as if one was expected to be cheerful and "keep one's chin up" all the time – there was no place for depression or tears. At times I became very frustrated and was then told I was being difficult and uncooperative. As shortage of staff and full wards was usually the norm, the nurses hadn't time for much individual attention and were always in a hurry. I hated being dressed untidily and left with my clothes twisted uncomfortably around my body, but if I mentioned it I was being fussy. Personal dignity is so very important at this time.'

It is not just a lack of counselling. There is no space allowed for us to express our grief and other emotions. Instead there is often pressure put on us to 'cope', and if we fail to live up to the standard demanded of us we are categorised as a 'problem'.

We often conform to the pressures to be 'strong'. Gina wrote: 'The emotional side was rather suffocated. Everyone kept saying how strong I was and that they were sure I could cope. It would have been good to have been encouraged to have had a good scream and cry instead of feeling guilty about breaking down. Everyone tried to be very jolly, which is probably essential, but there should be chances to discuss the future in more real terms.' Gina also made a remark which will strike a chord with many women: 'I often felt I was acting a role and keeping visitors at ease.'

Isabel, who was paralysed following a suicide attempt when she was 18, wrote, 'There was no one to talk to. Family and friends were in shock I think – and we were all busy glossing over the cause, pretending it was an accident. This was abroad – after about six months of this I came to England to a spinal unit and spent about six months there before I left. Again, there was no one to talk to in confidence. In all this time I cried three times. The first time I was told "This isn't like you"; the second time I stopped myself as I could see it was upsetting a ward maid; the third time I was sent back from physio in disgrace. Tears were definitely out. I feel now that counselling is vital. Also I was never told the precise implications of my injury and was too afraid/ashamed to ask. The spinal ward was overworked and understaffed – staff just didn't have time to discuss things, especially in private.'

In our lonely isolated grief, it is often other newly injured women who are the only source of comfort. As Claire put it: 'The only understanding of personal feelings came from the other women who were probably just as scared as me and communication was more of a knowing look or sigh to show the disparity of it all . . . Group discussions would have been a good idea.'

Most of us were left alone to deal with our feelings, although some talked of being able to 'open up' to a particular physio or occupational therapist. There was a common wish to be able to share experiences with, and learn from, other women. Libby summed up her experience. 'You couldn't talk to the staff about how you felt emotionally. It seems as if they deliberately ignored this side of things. I was able to talk to other patients, and the support we gave each other and the relationships that were formed is the main thing that made life bearable.'

One particular difficulty highlighted was that of getting

advice and support about sexual relationships. Thirty years ago, 19-year-old Valerie spent two years in a spinal unit and found 'there was no one to talk to about sexual hang-ups and fears about the future'. Beth, also injured in the 1950s, was told that she could have children but nothing was ever said about sex – a common experience. Things had not improved by 1981 when Amanda, who felt that, generally, her treatment was very good, complained that the subject of sexual relationships was neglected. 'I felt I could not talk to *anyone* about sexual feelings.'

Although the 'stiff upper lip' attitude adopted at most hospitals and spinal units did have one or two supporters, the overwhelming message was that women wanted, and needed, a more realistic and understanding approach. Andrea, for instance, wrote of the way that 'you were not supposed to feel unhappy or frustrated' and Alix explained how those who showed their feelings were regarded as 'soft'.

Getting to grips with basic emotional, as well as physical, problems is vital preparation for a life of disability. Unfortunately, most of us were not helped to get to grips with our emotions during our period of hospitalisation. Indeed, at a time when we desperately needed emotional support and practical help in coping with our new lives, many of us were thrown back almost entirely on our own resources. Annie was only 18 when she became a tetraplegic in 1978. She wrote: 'I was made to feel that I had to be strong and protect everyone from my grief, my family for their sake and nurses because they couldn't really help so I should not share it with them. I couldn't talk about my feelings anyway because I didn't want to admit them to myself. I was devastated by what had happened and spent all my time in a state of shock. I felt very alienated, even from myself. I didn't think others knew just how much I was suffering and yet could still appear "alright". It was just too horrific. I had lost everything, including my partner, career, house and car. I don't think enough emphasis was put on the emotional tragedy. Also, there was not enough information on benefits, entitlements or grants for alteration, etc. This was especially bad as it's probably the last thing you can think of for yourself. I felt that I needed someone to take over all those worries for me.'

No room for women?

Most of us were cynical about the overwhelming emphasis in spinal units on sport, competition and physical achievement, which left little room for our own concerns. Liz wrote: 'There was not enough emphasis on practical skills and personal care but too much emphasis on sport and walking and on cultivating competitive attitudes.' This over-emphasis seemed to be directly related to the rehabilitation programmes being geared primarily towards men with spinal cord injuries.

Rosalind also felt that there was too much emphasis on the physical achievement of, for example, walking with calipers at the expense of the emotional consequences of spinal cord injury. 'There wasn't anyone I could talk to about my feelings, and I used to find the constant jokiness and stiff upper lip attitude of the staff (and patients too) a strain. I sometimes felt I was pushed too hard in physiotherapy when I was exhausted, and there was too much emphasis on mastering walking with calipers. In fact, a bad fall while walking three days before I was due to be discharged delayed my discharge for six weeks.'

We often felt that we were pushed into an approach to physical achievement which we found oppressive – and inappropriate. Blanche wrote: 'Excellent though the physiotherapy was, I did find later that my performance improved with exercises done to music and for pleasure. Most things were sport-orientated. I hate competition and have no eye for balls or arrows.'

Matters of concern to women were neglected. As Helen put it, 'I have always felt that the rehabilitation programme ignored women's matters totally.' And Linda commented: 'the assumption was that the only thing wrong was paraplegia. It was difficult to get help with migraine or gynaecolog-

ical needs.' Part of this neglect of women's concerns arises
from women always being in a minority in a spinal unit, and
in fact June had the distressing experience of being the only
woman on the ward. 'I felt like a misplaced person, who had
to be tolerated,' she wrote. Gillian said: 'Never did I see
another young woman who had been through the hospital.
There was no one to talk to who had experienced the
trauma and who could pass things on to me or just to listen
while I poured out the feelings which I felt I couldn't tell
parents and work colleagues.'

The quality of care

The lack of attention to the emotional experience of paralysis often results in poorer quality care generally. Although
some stressed the high quality of the care received, many of
us had distressing experiences as a result of poor communication on the part of consultants, doctors and nurses. Often
this poor practice started right at the beginning, in that
women were not told they were permanently paralysed or
this fact was left untold until very late on. Sometimes we
were left to find out for ourselves. Geraldine, who was 13 at
the time of her accident, said, 'I was kept very much in the
dark about my condition and the extent of my injuries.
When I finally realised what my injuries were, I was left
alone to come to terms with it.'

Magda commented: 'In fact to this day the consultant has
never talked to me about my injury. I learnt through listening to what he told visiting doctors about me and looking at
my X-rays when he showed these to the visiting doctors.' It
is very common for doctors and consultants to behave as if
we had no right, or wish, to know about our injuries and the
consequences. Andrea summed up the experience of the
ward round when she said 'you were discussed as if you
were an idiot'.

A lack of communication is part of the generally power-
less situation in which we are placed in our relationships
with the professionals, and this is very much associated with

a poor standard of care. This is strikingly illustrated by Molly's experience. She started to develop numb patches when she was 17 in 1965 and then had a number of operations as a result of the spinal tumour which was then discovered. 'The emphasis while I was in hospital, of course, was on trying to remove the tumour, or at least giving it more space to grow by removing bone from the vertebrae. I was never told in the early stages that I could end up paralysed and in a wheelchair. I just assumed that I would get better. When I didn't and in fact got worse, and returned for more operations, there was no one to talk to about my feelings, even though after the last operation I came out of hospital in a wheelchair, having gone in with only a walking stick. I was never sent to a spinal unit for help or guidance. I feel I should have been – just to talk to others and learn how to use a wheelchair properly.'

Hospitals seem to have given very little thought to the needs of individual patients in terms of timing and type of information. Bridget felt that a cruel trick was played on her as a result of this. 'I knew immediately after my accident that I was permanently paralysed but, in the first few days of grief and terror, a doctor told me that I would probably walk again. In retrospect I think that the hospital had a policy of not telling you anything until the shock of the accident had worn off, but the effect was to make things more difficult for me in that he gave me unwarranted hope. Things were also made worse by the fact that the nurses initially did not believe that I had fallen while trying to rescue a child but seemed to think that I had attempted suicide. They behaved in a very cool manner towards me until the story appeared in the local press.'

Fiona, a doctor herself, was paralysed after an unnecessary operation for a (wrongly) suspected recurrent tumour. She wrote, 'There was appalling communication in the neurological unit. People avoided me. No one would say that I was having any difficulty. I really think they hoped that I would die as I was an embarrassment. The day I was moved to the younger disabled unit, the neurosurgeon said that he would come to see me in 10 days, and that I would be walking (he did not come!). This was about seven weeks after my operation.'

Cecily experienced additional traumas because of a failure to diagnose her spinal cord injury. She had been working as a school meals supervisor and slipped on hot fat spilt on the floor at work. She felt numb down one side but was sent home from hospital without anyone considering that she might have damaged her spinal cord. 'After five weeks I was, if anything, in a worse condition and eventually my doctor made an appointment for me to see a specialist who ordered physiotherapy. This made me even worse.' It was not until six months after her accident that injury to the spinal cord was diagnosed. The whole experience was made worse by poor communication. She continued: 'Injury to my neck was only found when in desperation I consulted a neurosurgeon privately, needing to know for myself why I was experiencing certain things and getting no answers from the hospital doctors who, it was apparent, had no idea of what I was experiencing or any understanding of how I felt.'

The tragedy of poor communication practice is that good communication can make such a difference to how we are able to cope. Denise is one of the few women who felt that her doctor positively helped her in this way: 'He explained so well about my body and what I should expect.' Madeline also had nothing but praise for her consultant: 'We had a brilliant doctor in charge of our ward, who would explain anything you asked about, and who always asked how things had gone after a weekend at home, how the children had reacted, etc.'

Unfortunately, it was more common to experience a general lack of attention to emotional needs and this often prompted criticism of the care provided. Claire spoke for many of us when she wrote: 'The physio and OT [occupational therapist] were excellent but on the ward far too much time was spent making us obey stupid unnecessary rules . . . Many of us were treated like third-class citizens and a lot of us were totally stripped of personal dignity.'

Spinal units often operated fairly rigid procedures which, as Linda wrote, were 'too inflexible to cater specifically for individual needs. The assumption that you should conform to the norm of a 48-hour bowel pattern led to considerable distress . . . Bladder training left me for up to two hours at a time in a pool of urine which developed a skin weakness which remains an ongoing problem.'

Bladder training was also a problem for Marion, 51 at the time of her accident, who felt that the nurses did not take account of the fact that some patients were older and weaker than others. 'When it came to bladder training this was my hardest time. I always felt too much trouble and was very reluctant to ask for help. Having a weak voice did not help. There were times when no one took any notice of me.'

With regard to the quality of care, as well as for all other aspects of our experience of hospitalisation, many of us recognised that a shortage of resources was often at the root of the problem. Martha, injured in 1984, wrote that going to her spinal unit 'was like going back 50 years in time. But my spinal unit doesn't have Jimmy Savile to raise funds and public attention. The treatment was as good as the health service allows – there were often too few nurses for patients. I learned why patients are called such – because [patience is] the most important thing to learn in order to keep your sanity.'

What about the future?

The failure of most hospitals and spinal units to address our emotional needs inevitably led to difficulties in getting help to make decisions about our future. Most of us spend months in hospital, and while there we have to make preparations for picking up our lives again. As with other aspects of our experience of hospitalisation, there is remarkable similarity in the concerns expressed by women injured over the last 30 years.

Eileen, who became a tetraplegic in 1961 at the age of 14, said, 'I left hospital feeling that wiping a wet flannel around my face and shovelling food into my mouth was all I'd ever be able to do. I was never given any real hope or real advice for the future. No one suggested I returned to school or tried to find work.' Margery was also injured in 1961. She was three months pregnant at the time of her car accident and felt that 'while treatment was alright in the early stages, there was little explanation and no discussion of the future. I was worried about the effect on my unborn baby and the ability to cope with a young family.'

Wendy broke her neck when she fell down a flight of stairs at home in 1981. She wrote: 'I felt very lonely and cut off in hospital despite regular family and friends visiting. Also, no one asked the patients if plans made on their behalf for the future were suitable or right for them. I had the feeling of being "steam rollered" along without proper consultation by hospital or community social workers.'

Louise identified the kind of help she would have appreciated after her accident in 1985. 'I would have liked to have been informed about other aspects of my new life, e.g. problems with compensation claims, problems with local authorities, problems with access, and emotional and psychological problems. I would have liked to have been put in touch with paraplegics of much longer standing to find out how one can cope in the long term.'

Part of the difficulty in getting help with planning our future is that hospital professionals seem to have a very limited view of our abilities. This is illustrated by Bridget's experience after her accident in 1983. 'I discovered that, although the consultant had told me I would be able to return to my job and to looking after my 1-year-old daughter, he changed his tune once he found out that I was a single parent. His assumptions about my potential for "independence" seemed in fact to be based on the idea that I would have a husband to be dependent upon. Once he found out that I didn't, the question was raised as to whether I could (at the age of 33!) go back and live with my parents.' It seems that in general the health and social services professionals have little concept of enabling us to return to our lives as they were before injury; instead, they have stereotypical ideas of passive roles for us. They see us as being cared for by husbands or parents. This is particularly ironic as the evidence from the questionnaires is that women, who tend to be the primary carers within their families before injury, in fact return to their caring role after injury. Such assumptions on the part of professionals also have very serious implications for single women, as it means they are more likely to end up in residential care. (This is discussed in Chapter 4.)

Conclusion

Of the 205 women who responded to our questionnaire, a small minority praised the treatment they received during the long months in hospital. The majority, however, found that communication of the vital information about paralysis was poor; that their emotional experience was ignored; that their needs as women were not addressed; and finally that they were given little help in planning for the future. This experience seems to be as common in the 1980s as it was during the 1950s, 1960s and 1970s. It was certainly one of the strongest messages to come from the Women's Conferences held by the SIA.

3.

Our Daily Lives

This chapter deals with daily living and what makes this possible for us. The issue of whether or not we have sufficient resources to meet our additional needs runs through all sections of this chapter. Disability brings with it increased costs, particularly if we are to return to independent living. At the same time our earning power and that of our families is threatened. In many ways, an inability to meet the increased costs has a more dramatic and fundamental effect on our lives than the disability itself.

A place to live

When an accident or illness suddenly causes paralysis, our lives stand still and many months (sometimes years) go by before we can start to take up the threads again. One of the most important barriers to be overcome is that which is created when we find, after injury, that our homes are no longer accessible to us. Whether we are single, married, with or without children, a home is the pivot on which the rest of our life depends; something taken for granted until, because of our paralysis, it becomes a place that we can no longer enter and move around in unaided. The step at the front door which previously we did not even notice now becomes an obstacle which renders us helpless; a flight of stairs takes half our home away; and the size and layout of the kitchen and bathroom may make it impossible to do things that we did not think twice about doing before.

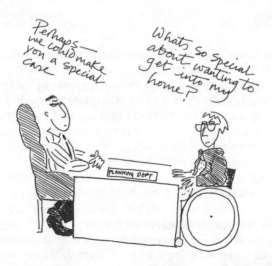

The availability of suitable housing is a most important factor in what way, and, indeed, whether, we return to pick up the threads of our lives again. For those whose level of disability means that physically accessible housing has also to be combined with personal care, the obstacles are even greater.

Some of us never achieve independent living again. This was the experience of both Antonia and Adela. Antonia, from Portugal, was injured at the level of C4, 5 and 6 in her early 20s. On leaving the spinal unit she writes, 'I had no option but to go into residential care as I have no family in England. I'm not happy to be living here. I want my individuality to be recognised and appreciated. I want my own home where I am boss.'

Adela also had to enter residential care when she found the strain of trying to find accessible accommodation too much. Following a minor heart attack during the search she gave in to the pressure put upon her to seek residential care. Aged 67 and a widow at the time of her paralysis, she writes, 'It was a great wrench to give up my home which my husband and I had furnished together, my personal possessions and the garden, and to say goodbye to my friends and neighbours.'

Suitable housing is very important in enabling us to return to independent living. However, from the experience of the women taking part in this project, a crucial factor in this return is whether we are single or married/cohabiting at the time of injury. Single women, whatever their age or level of injury, are more likely to end up in residential care and this is a damning indictment of current housing and social services provided, or, rather, not provided, as there is no need for these women to lose their independence. As Bridget put it, 'The professions seem to be dominated by the idea that independent living is only viable if you have a husband (or possibly parents) to be dependent upon. This is nonsense, but it can lead to women not being given the help they need to return to their lives before their injury.'

Ten women went into residential care on leaving hospital; seven were tetraplegic and two (one of whom was also tetraplegic) were aged 60 or over at the time of injury. However, age and level of disability do not by any means determine whether we have to go into residential care. Five women who took part in this project were over 60 at the time of their injury, one a tetraplegic and the other four low paraplegic wheelchair users (that is, T7 or below). Two of these women were single (one of them widowed) at the time of their injury and both went into residential care. The other three, who were all married, returned to their own homes.

The link between marriage/cohabitation and being able to return home is also clear when we look at the women between the ages of 16 and 59. Only one of the 92 married or cohabiting women in this age group went into residential care. On the other hand, of the 97 single women in the same age group, seven went into residential care.

Again, amongst tetraplegic women, it is the lack of a partner to aid the return home which is linked to residential care. None of the 13 married or cohabiting women who were tetraplegic went into residential care, while seven of the 31 single tetraplegic women did. Age and level of disability do not inevitably prevent us from returning to an independent life, neither, in spite of the importance of having a partner, does being single condemn us to institutional care, as the majority of single women do in fact return to independent living. However, the link between having a partner and being able to return to our own homes shows up the inadequacy of the statutory services in meeting the needs of those of us who cannot look to our families or partners to provide support. It is the lack of enabling resources, rather than disability, which creates dependence.

Anita's experience highlights this particular failure. Paralysed in 1967 at the level of C5/6 when she was single and aged 25, her expectations of being able to 'go back into the community, with some help from all the various agencies and find a job back in nursing' were soon dashed. 'I found,' she wrote, 'that there was nowhere I could live, no help at hand when I needed it. And, as a tetraplegic, nobody actually wanted you in a job. It was like being a total write off by society. A reject overnight. I went into residential care, through no choice of my own, sentenced without committing a crime.' Her mother was not able to cope with having her at home as her father had died suddenly the month before her accident. Anita did not want to become dependent on her mother anyway, but 'Nobody knew what to do with me so I was consigned to live my days out in institutional care'.

After spending 10 years 'existing' in various institutions she met her husband (who is also disabled) and together they fought to achieve independent housing, eventually setting up one of the first independent living schemes in the country. 'My life changed totally from "existing" to living a more fulfilled life within my capacity. I feel angry and upset at those 10 wasted years, like an innocent prisoner must feel.'

Some of us in our 20s and 30s when injured found that a return to our parents' home was the only course of action offered when we left hospital. Rosalind had left her parents' home 10 years before she was knocked down by a lorry at the age of 32. She had been living in a privately rented flat at the top of a Victorian terraced house. 'Not only were there steps to the front door and then three flights of stairs to my flat but the bathroom was up yet another flight of stairs. I never went back there which was very upsetting.'

She went to live with her parents after leaving the spinal

unit. Their house was not fully accessible, which made her dependent on her mother and the district nurse, and made life more difficult than it need have been. 'I found it very difficult being completely reliant on my parents again,' she wrote, 'having lived independently for more than 10 years. It almost felt like reverting to childhood again and I think for a while they treated me differently. It made me feel more disabled than I was. I realised that it was difficult for them, too.'

Significantly, Rosalind did not even consider looking for accommodation in the private sector – private tenancies accessible to wheelchair users do not exist, and she could not at that point afford to buy a property. Her only source of independent housing was the local council, who nominated her to a housing association specialising in housing for disabled people.

Twenty-six women, who had previously lived in their own homes, found that a return to their parents' home was the only option offered following injury. Ten are high level paraplegic or tetraplegic wheelchair users and only two were married at the time of injury. A lack of financial and practical support from anywhere else forced Amanda, for example, at the age of 24, to live with her parents when she became a C6 tetraplegic. 'I didn't want to go back home after leading an independent life,' she wrote, yet there was no alternative. Later her independence was re-established when an extension was built so that she now has 'independence and freedom, but help is close at hand, which is comforting'.

Lynne's experience demonstrates how much independence can be gained, even with a high level of injury, when the housing and personal care are provided to suit our needs. Paralysed from the shoulders down at the age of 18, with little use of her hands, Lynne nevertheless returned to university, completed postgraduate study in the USA, and now works full-time and lives on her own. All this was made possible by the right type of housing combined with personal care. She currently lives in a housing co-op flat, and employs three neighbours to help her get up in the morning and go to bed at night.

During the long months in hospital, we somehow have to plan for when we get home. Most of us return to the home that we left, and find we either have to have alterations done or find somewhere more suitable. Coming back home can be upsetting, as Charlotte found when she returned to her parents' home after her car accident when she was 17. 'When I first came home I felt alienated because of having been away so long. It was a funny feeling, like being a stranger in one's own home which one had grown up in. The early frustrations were intense.'

On the other hand, Harriet drew strength from being able to return to her family's house. Her father worked very hard to make their home (up-country in Nigeria) accessible to her. She writes, 'My own Dad paid for everything and I should confess it was actually taxing for him as we are not well off. I was very glad with the fact that I was able to manage in our own simple home without any problem. It was really encouraging to me when I faced no problems living there with my own family.'

Only 26 women moved straight from hospital into new accommodation suitable for their needs, seven of these to purpose-built housing, the others to adapted housing. Nine of us returned to new homes which had not been adapted. Most of us, a total of 128, returned to our previous homes (our own or our parents') although 21 then found we had to move house within two years. The difficulty of finding suitable accommodation and/or doing alterations often means that we have to stay in hospital longer than necessary. We do not appear in the homeless statistics because our homelessness is hidden, but this is nevertheless a real experience. Ellen, for example, spent seven-and-a-half months longer than necessary in hospital (14 months altogether), 'simply because a suitable home had to be acquired and altered to suit my disability.' One hundred and twenty-eight of us were in hospital for seven months or longer, and 44 in hospital over a year.

The desire to take up our lives again often drives us to return to unsuitable housing and adds to our dependence on others. Ninety-four of us expressed dissatisfaction with our housing when we came out of hospital (although only 13 are still not happy). Many had to turn a living or dining room into a bedroom and to rely on help to get to inaccessible bathrooms and toilets. Theresa lived for 18 months 'unable to get into the kitchen and frontwards, only on to the loo. I needed two district nurses to help me into the bath.' The alterations that were finally made – installation of a lift, adapted kitchen, widened doorways with sliding doors, adapted bathroom, central heating and carport – made her life possible again.

For Louise, injured in 1985 and still awaiting compensation, life is impossible. 'My house is completely unsuitable for me but no alterations are possible. I cannot get in and out of the front door without help. I have only access to the downstairs front and back rooms. No access to the kitchen. No access to the garden. No access to the bedroom. No access to the toilet and bathroom. I have to rely on my husband for everyday care on a 24-hour basis. I feel angry beyond words about the housing situation. I am more handicapped than I need be because of it. My relationship with my husband and children is strained. I suffer from a lot of depression.'

Nadine's house was also inaccessible to her, but with council grants, insurance money and an interim compensation award she was able to do the necessary adaptations. 'The common sense action would have been to sell the house and buy a bungalow, but as we had spent almost all our married life here and our friends and neighbours were so supportive, we chose to stay . . . I feel that when your whole life has been changed you hang on to familiar things.'

Often our homes cannot be adapted and we have to seek somewhere else to live. For those able to do so, the necessity of moving home can be an upsetting experience, adding to the feeling that our lives have been shattered by paralysis. The majority of the new homes, although more suitable, still have to have alterations done. It is assumed that bungalows are the most appropriate form of housing for us (if we are lucky enough to live in an area where there are any), but often it is not as simple as that. Most bungalows still have steps to the front and back doors – or thresholds that are six inches high; toilets and bathrooms are often inaccessible because of their size or layout; and kitchens will not necessarily be big enough. There are other reasons which may render them unsuitable. Hannah's local council could only offer a two-bedroom bungalow – and suggested that one of her children should live with a relative. She insisted that instead they adapt her house to enable her to remain there and look after her children.

For most of us it is the availability of money, or of council grants or council or housing association properties, which determine whether or not we can get the housing we need. Theresa's experience confirms how important money is. The adaptations which were made possible by her compensation released her from dependence on her mother, enabled her to look after her three children, and to survive a painful divorce. She is a C7/8 tetraplegic and writes: 'I lead a completely independent life.'

Adapting a property, even a bungalow, can be expensive. It can also take a long time to find something suitable and to have the work done. Helen writes of how 'it took a lot of visits to find a bungalow with three bedrooms, suitable layout and within our price range. It was necessary to relocate the front door, enlarge and refit the kitchen and bathroom and provide front and rear ramps and install central heating.' These alterations were made possible by the local authority grant of £14,000 (in 1984) which she was lucky enough to obtain with little difficulty.

Unfortunately, a more common experience of obtaining grants from local councils is that they take ages to get, are often not enough and, for some items which we would consider essential, are not available at all. Injured in 1983, Marion and her husband paid for alterations themselves as 'we were told by the local council that they had run out of money and we would have to wait'.

Another possible solution to our housing problems is to turn to the local council or housing associations to provide rented accommodation. We are one of the groups of people most dramatically affected by the diminishing supply of council accommodation as, except for those of us lucky enough to get compensation, we are very unlikely to have the economic resources to pay for the sudden large housing costs made necessary by our disability. In spite of the cut-backs in council housing, the majority of disabled people still look to the public rented sector to solve their housing problems.

Perhaps the last word on housing should go to 27-year-old Martha, whose nomadic attitude to life has not been changed by her paraplegia. She was injured when travelling in the USA, and while hospitalised in Britain applied to 'dozens of housing authorities, trusts, councils, co-ops'. She got nowhere with any of them and returned to live with her parents for a while. She writes: 'My parents' place was in an isolated country location where little was accessible but the views were beautiful. I now live in Manhattan New York where the reverse is true.' She goes on to say, 'My place is not permanent but I don't want to be permanent. The idea of a fixed house seems very limiting to me. As long as I can get my chair through the bathroom door and up alongside the loo and bath I can live anywhere.'

Personal care

Personal care is an issue for us, as paralysis means that we can no longer take for granted the routine things of daily life. All of us require at least some alterations in our physical sur-roundings to enable us to be independent, and some need help from other people. We have complicated feelings about receiving help; on the one hand helpers can bring about independence, on the other their very necessity can make us feel helpless and dependent.

Only 43 of us did not need any help when we first came out of hospital. For the rest who did need help by far the most common source was family (not including partners/ husbands) or friends (for 56 women). Partners/husbands provided personal care for another 19, outside agencies (dis-trict nurses, home helps, etc.) for 26, while 49 women relied on a combination of all three. Ten women went into residential care on leaving hospital. By the time they came to answer the questionnaire, 44 women who initially had had help with personal care found they no longer needed it, while 36 needed less. Fifty-nine women reported that they relied on the same amount of help as previously, and 6 women required more help than before.

For those women who do need help with day-to-day living, the level and type of assistance varies according to both physical and social circumstances. For some high level tetraplegics every physical movement requires help – from eating and drinking to managing bladders and bowels. For other tetraplegics, a high level of independence is achieved by maximising the use of the arms. For a paraplegic, personal care needs are determined by whether it is possible to transfer into and out of the wheelchair unaided, or whether the wheelchair can be lifted into a car without help, and so on. Whatever level of injury sustained, our physical abilities will be directly related to whether or not we received the specialist treatment we needed at a spinal unit. Regardless of our physical abilities, however, if we live in unsuitable housing, where the toilet is upstairs or the kitchen down a flight of stairs, for example, our level of dependence on others will be higher than it need be.

Since few of us relied on others for help with daily living before we were paralysed, it is not surprising that our initial reaction is frustration and guilt about being dependent. Some of us continue to hate this feature of our lives. Hannah 'did not like the idea of being dependent on others' when she first became paralysed at the age of 32. Now, five years later, she writes: 'I am still in the same situation and still hate being dependent on other people and I get very frustrated.'

Rebecca, who became paraplegic as a result of a motor bike accident when she was 27 years old, spoke for many when she said, 'I felt just like a child at first, having to be carried up and down stairs. It was frustrating for me.' However, she was lucky in that this situation only lasted a short time before she moved into a bungalow where the adaptations which her husband carried out enabled her to be independent.

Helen writes of the embarrassment she felt in 'having to involve other people in dealing with the most personal things for me'. Now, an adapted bungalow and aids such as a self-propelled shower chair enable her to manage with very little help, and indeed she has returned to being the primary carer in her family. She writes: 'Our adapted bungalow is very well equipped for me as a housewife and mother of two daughters.'

Molly also had young children when she became a wheelchair user and, when she first returned home, like Helen she found it difficult to rely on others for personal care. She writes: 'I needed help to get in and out of the bath and hated it. I also needed "turning over" at night and helping to the loo. My dignity was hurt and I felt clumsy, ugly and repulsive.' Her gradual return to independence, made possible by aids and adapted housing, enables her now to say, 'I feel more free and independent here because we have learned how to make things more convenient and so my confidence has increased as a result.'

Anger is an emotion which can become bound up with personal care issues. Pauline, who became a tetraplegic at the age of 34, writes, 'One of the biggest problems at home is the high frustration level. It is hard to accept that things would not be done as I would have done them – housework, cooking, ironing, even hanging washing on the line, which might sound petty but it can really get to you. Even now, I sit with friends while they do things and I'm always one step ahead; at times they look so hamfisted and I can see an easier way, but I'm learning to bite my tongue. Sheer frustration at not being able to help gets out of proportion at times. It doesn't always seem to get easier. It helps to talk about it but I didn't expect to experience so much anger towards myself because I can't do my share.'

For those who have to rely on statutory services for personal care, the frustrations of having to fit into the district/ community nurse's routine can also be great. Norma, injured at the level of C6 when she was 17, wrote, 'We did have a district nurse call but by the time she arrived in the mornings it was almost 12 o'clock, so my mother or sisters

would get me up and dress me long before she turned up.'
Her complaints about the district nurse's timetable are
echoed by 12 other women. It is for this reason that Nora's
mother took on all her daughter's personal care. Nora
remembers her unhappiness at being dependent on her
mother at the age of 21. 'There was a feeling of frustration
and resentment being wholly dependent on others – nothing
can ever be done quite as you want it yourself. Also, I felt
that no part of my life, not even the most personal, would
ever again be private.' However, she has now been paralysed over 20 years and writes, 'I realised eventually that I
had to accept the fact I was entirely dependent, otherwise I
couldn't get on with living. It has made a big difference since
my husband took over my personal care, especially as he
didn't know me before my accident and therefore accepts
me exactly as I am. Because we are very close and have a
sharing relationship, I now hardly notice that I can't do
these things myself. It's not an important issue any more.'

The loss of privacy when we need substantial personal
care can be exacerbated if we have to rely on strangers. We
may also find it difficult to ask others for help. Jackie wrote:
'When I first went home, I absolutely hated having to ask for
any help whatsoever. The district nurses at first were not
very forthcoming which made it worse. I found sometimes I
would do without rather than ask. Now I suppose I have
accepted the fact that I do need help and if I want to get on
with what I want to do and look the way I want to look I
have to ask people to do things for me. I now have different
district nurses who are a lot more helpful and I have a lot
more friends now who usually offer help before I have a
chance to ask.'

Vicky also found asking and accepting help very difficult
to begin with. 'I hated asking for help with anything. My
mother and I don't get on too well and my father is rather
shy. I preferred to take two hours to get dressed than get
help from mother. We got no help from district nurses – the
only time they came to change a catheter [a small tube
inserted into the urethra] they were so unimpressive I didn't
think to ask for help. Most things I just worked at until I

found a way of coping. Friends and relatives outside immediate family were so embarrassed by the whole situation that
it was easier not to ask for anything. I think this was wrong –
more ice is broken by action than just looking.' In fact, she
now says, 'I have found that people like being given specific
things to do, rather than just gazing at the wheelchair. Sur-
reptitiously passing a plate across for cutting up food in a
restaurant makes both of you feel as though you are sharing a secret, while if I just struggle with awkward dishes
on my own we are all embarrassed. It's the same with trans-
fers; if I give a spectator the armrest to hold he feels less
helpless and I am not hampered by the wrong sort of help. It
took me a long time to realise that I had to take the initia-
tive.'

For a few of us, circumstances have increased the dependence on others and isolation from the rest of the world.
Ellen was injured at the level of T12/L1 at the age of 34. Six
weeks after coming out of hospital to a new home, her
father died of cancer and three months later her husband
asked for a divorce. Her whole life had been centred on her
marriage, particularly as she worked in her husband's business which she had helped to build up. Ellen writes of how
she hated being dependent on others when she was first
paralysed but 'despite my strong feelings about dependence
on others, I have become more dependent over the years,
from nerves and fears, and a total lack of self confidence'.
She had little or no advice or support from statutory agencies and, after leaving the spinal unit, no contact with other
people with disabilities.

After her husband left, Ellen's mother came to live with
her – at which point her home help hours were reduced –
and Ellen has continued to be dependent on her mother
since then. She writes: 'I feel my paralysis demolished my
life completely. Also, other changes in my life which followed in its wake – mainly my divorce. I feel I have
achieved nothing, apart from existing from one day to the
next. I have become apathetic and totally disinterested with
living.' Like many of us she feels she has not lived up to
others' expectations and writes: 'I am a failed paraplegic.'

Ellen's lack of support from statutory or voluntary agencies helps to create both her and her mother's isolation. Her dependence increases her vulnerability to any change in her circumstances, for instance, if her mother becomes ill or dies.

It is our material situations and resources (primarily, whether or not we have an adequate income) which essentially determine the quality of our lives. This is evident in our experiences of finding suitable housing, and also in our attempts to meet our needs for personal care. Those of us who have waged work, or whose partners or parents do, and those of us who receive compensation for our injury will find it easier to live independent lives than those who do not.

Eighty-two of us have to pay for private help with care and/or housework. Lynne, for example, uses a combination of financial help from her local Social Services/Attendance Allowance and her own salary to pay for the carers which make her independent life as a tetraplegic possible. She is particularly happy with the fact that she is responsible for employing her carers as such a relationship can be fragile. 'It has taken me a long time to be able to choose the right people and to get the "carer relationship" working. It is a very tricky relationship – a lot of it is luck, but most is building up a mutually acceptable situation for both people by respecting each other's situations, listening to each other's needs and being totally honest about what one likes and dislikes.'

Lynne employs three neighbours as carers. Anita also looks to her local community for finding paid carers. 'For personal help since I have moved out of an institution I have always asked the local community to help and have always had a good response. I think I am fortunate because I live in a close supportive mining community. Usually my helpers are just ordinary folks with no training. They come with no preconceptions and form much healthier relationships with me than anyone who has had even a mild breather at the local hospital. With the folks that are willing to learn we are able to have a far more equal relationship than anyone trying to tell me what is best for me.'

Anita now also has a Home Care Aide provided by the local Social Services Department who helps to cook meals, etc. 'I used to do this myself, but since I got so involved in local politics, health groups and other things I have been exhausted. The Home Care Aide was specially requested so that I could be actively involved in the community rather than being tied to home.'

Valerie is another tetraplegic who spent many years in residential care but who now lives independently. 'I could not bear depending on help and this drove me to making myself independent,' she wrote. 'I now manage all my own personal care and have designed clothes that make dressing easier. I use a suppository inserter to assist bowel care.' This aid has in fact enabled many tetraplegics to be independent in a most important way.

Barbara, also a tetraplegic, uses the same aid and is also able to be generally independent in personal care but finds that the 'relentlessness of all the routines, day in, day out' and the time that it takes to get herself dressed, etc. make life very difficult with a full-time job. She therefore chooses to rely on her mother to help with personal care – 'I could not manage to work full-time and look after myself.'

Our own role as carers within our families usually continues after injury, and, indeed, many women measure the 'success' or otherwise of their return to independent living in terms of whether or not they are still able to look after their families.

Other women, whether married or single, have gained strength from recognising that they would rather use the help of others in day-to-day living which has then enabled them to spend time and energy on working outside the home, on political activity, in community involvement or leisure activities. Unfortunately, the health and social services professionals very rarely see us as other than merely passive recipients of other people's caring services.

Transport

Following our paralysis, if we are not to be confined to our own homes, we have to rely on transport of some kind to enable us to work, to ferry our children about, to have a social or political life. Most of us have to accept that buses and the underground are inaccessible, with the exception of someone like Helen who lives close to the Tyne and Wear Metro which is fully accessible for wheelchair users, or Geraldine who says 'In my city we have a corporation bus that has a chair lift on the side'. Why cannot all buses have one?

Cars become the most important form of transport. We are therefore dependent either on our own economic resources or schemes such as Dial-a-Ride. An absence of either restricts our lives and increases our dependence on others. Seventy-four of us cannot drive and six of us can drive but do not have a car. Sandra, for instance, cannot afford a car and there is no Dial-a-Ride in her area. Her independence has been slightly increased, however, by the gift of a Batricar from her local technical college. The restrictions which she experiences as a result of not being able to afford a car illustrate how important an adequate income is for independent living.

Batricars, or other outdoor battery-driven wheelchairs or scooters, can greatly increase our freedom of movement and are very useful for local trips. They are, however, very expensive to buy, costing over £1,000 and are rarely available through health or social services departments.

Nicola, paralysed when she was still at school but now working as a clerk typist, writes, 'Being able to drive and having my own transport means the world to me. I have freedom and independence. I can go wherever I please, within reason. I travel to and from work each day.'

Those of us who were issued with 'trikes', the blue three-wheelers now discontinued and replaced with mobility allowance, have mixed feelings about them. To some, the possession of such a vehicle spelt independence. Beth, injured in 1955 when she was 14 years old, got a 'ministry three-wheeler' as soon as she was 17. 'My parents didn't have a car, nor would they push the wheelchair in public so for two years I didn't get about much unless friends helped.'

To others, however, the isolation of a car which would only take one person added to our difficulties. Ellen wrote of her 'trike': 'I kept it for three years but lost confidence and hated being alone in the vehicle. I returned it. I have not driven since so I use taxis and, recently, Dial-a-Ride.' She comments how the introduction of Dial-a-Ride has made transport easier and less expensive, echoing the praise of many of us who are lucky enough to have such a scheme in our area.

Celia, who drives her own car, nevertheless also finds Dial-a-Ride invaluable because of the difficulties of finding somewhere to park. Insurmountable parking problems, together with general access problems, were in fact responsible for her having to give up her job.

When Valerie was first paralysed in 1955 it was unheard of for a tetraplegic like herself to drive. She became one of the first tetraplegics to gain this form of independence when she passed her test 13 years after her injury. She can now say, 'Transport is not too big a problem for me.'

Some of us qualified for a 'Ministry Mini' as disabled mothers. Molly was quite happy with hers, although it took nine months to get one. Karen had to prove to the Artificial Limbs and Appliances Centre (ALAC) that 'it was physically impossible to put a baby into a carrycot in a mini saloon from a wheelchair. I was then given a clubman estate.' And Pamela also had problems with bureaucracy: ' . . . the social worker at [the spinal unit] forgot to send the form in so it was a year and a near breakdown before I got it. Plus they never told me I need not retake my test so it was another six months before I was out and about driving.'

The importance of seeing what other disabled people can do is illustrated by Jemma's experience. Injured in 1955 she writes, 'I bought a car straight away and learnt to drive it. This was thanks to an older paraplegic who came to see me having heard about me. He arrived in a Morris Minor with all the hand controls, and I was absolutely amazed that anyone could drive when paralysed. So I ordered a car and had it fitted with hand controls.'

Most of us require very minor adaptations to a car in order to drive: an automatic gear box, hand controls (which are very simple, cost about £100 and take 30 minutes to fit) and sometimes a knob on the steering wheel to make turning it with one hand easier. The more difficult question is how to get the wheelchair in the car if we don't want to rely on someone else to do this for us.

Those of us who go to spinal units are more likely to have had advice from physiotherapists on how to get a wheelchair into the car without help, and the ability to do this greatly adds to our independence. We can still achieve this independence if we are able to afford one of the various electrical solutions on the market, for example, a mechanism which lifts the wheelchair into a box on the roof of the car. Or the Car Chair (an electric wheelchair which is lifted electrically into the car and becomes the driver's, or passenger's, seat) which Ingrid bought and of which she writes, 'Now I have a Car Chair, I am completely independent.'

Some tetraplegics, such as Samantha, have had their mobility greatly increased through buying a car such as the Chairman Metro which takes both her and her wheelchair so that she does not have to transfer into a car seat. However, such vehicles (and the equipment mentioned in the previous paragraph) are expensive and Samantha used money raised by her friends to buy one. As a passenger rather than a driver, and as a single parent, Samantha also has to rely on the availability of Care Attendants to drive her. She is lucky in that there is a Community Service Volunteer scheme in her area. If there were no Care Attendants or Independent Living Scheme she would find transport a major problem.

Public transport for us is mainly restricted to trains and planes. We have a diverse experience of both the accessibility of British Rail and airports and the attitude of the staff. Travelling in the guard's van on a cold day in January can be a horrific experience; on the other hand, to travel first class at a reduced fare can sometimes be very pleasant. As Martha says, 'Being disabled brings out the best and the worst in people' and whether the journey is a pleasure or not depends to a large extent on the arbitrary nature of British Rail staffs' attitudes towards us.

The same goes for airports. As Beth put it (writing in 1985), 'Heathrow is very obstructive – no one is responsible for a wheelchair passenger, it seems, when you arrive at the terminal, whereas Gatwick are very helpful, even to lone travellers in chairs.' Belinda was once put on a fork lift truck in order to get on to a plane but does not let such an experience, or the fact that she cannot drive, deter her from her love of travel. She has been to Borneo three times since her injury and only wishes that coaches had a part at the back for a wheelchair which would allow her to go on continental coach tours.

Daily living

As women, part of our return to 'normal' life is often a return to the pressures of looking after other people. Aids and adaptations which are supposedly about helping us to be independent are in fact often about enabling others to be dependent on us for the tasks which keep a house clean and a family fed. Society's expectations of women being what they are, it is not surprising that many of us measure our 'success' or 'failure' in terms of whether we can return to the role of housewife and mother.

Erica had a struggle to resume her role within her family because she is in constant pain. 'At first I found it very difficult to cope as I still hadn't learnt to override the pain factor. My GP was very supportive and together we worked out ways that meant I could cope at the right times during the day. His advice was: "So long as you can cheerfully wave your husband and children off in the morning and welcome them home with a real smile, the problems during the day are immaterial." From the start I attempted to use that advice and it has worked. It made me very happy to realise that the children regarded me as the same "Mum".'

Jeanette also describes how she returned to her role as wife and mother. 'It is very difficult to describe how I manage, but I cook and clean for four adults [her sons are grown up] and entertain friends quite often. So I suppose I must manage quite well. We streamlined the kitchen to cut out as much work as possible. I have a ceramic hob built into the worktop which makes movement of pans and cleaning easy. I work at a pull-out table top at right angles to the cooker. I have an automatic washer and can hang washing out on a rotary clothes line positioned on the patio just outside the kitchen door. I shop for small items at the village store but go for large weekly shops at the supermarket with my family.'

Tessa, paraplegic since the age of 20, has now married, works full-time and has the dual role which so many working married women have. She writes of her housework: 'I usually go shopping alone, by car. Our Sainsbury's has trolleys which attach to wheelchairs. My husband hoovers the main part of the carpets and dusts high shelves. I do the rest of the cleaning. I use a feather duster on a stick and a cylinder vacuum cleaner for the edges. I spent a long time looking for one which was powerful but light enough for me to lift – an Electrolux electronic. My cooking rings are 740 mm from the floor and are individual ones set into the work surface. The oven has a shelf the same height as a formica wheelchair tray my father made so I can slide heavy things in and out. I use a long handled little fork for weeding. Our flower beds are narrow.'

Whether we work outside the home, whether or not we live with a partner, the work which goes into the daily servicing of ourselves and/or others has to be done. Housework is an issue because it is something that most of us, whatever our situation, did before our injury and, if we cannot do it after paralysis, it is still often our responsibility to organise for someone else to do the work.

Rosalind, aged 32 and single at the time of her road accident, carried on as before, once she managed to get a flat of her own. 'When first injured, I did most of my own cleaning. It's possible to do a lot of housework sitting in a wheelchair, although it's difficult to do things like cleaning the bath, hoovering, cleaning the floors, making the bed. I used to do all my washing in the bath (just as I used to before my accident) until I bought a washing machine. Now, however, I do very little housework, partly because it's boring and I find it hard work, but also because I spend so much time on personal care. Doing things like having a bath takes up more time than before and if I still did all my housework I would have time for nothing else. I was starting to find that all the time I wasn't at work was taken up with personal care and housework and I had no time, or energy, to do anything else. Also, the home help service from the council is so good, which helps. I still do my ironing as the home help hours only cover shopping and cleaning, and I pay someone else to clean the windows.'

Some of us consciously resist the pressures to prove we can cope unaided. Anita is clear that her political and community involvement is more important to her than struggling to do household tasks. She writes, 'I did try and prove all sorts of things to myself and didn't call on the help I could have had. Over the years I have realised that involvement in matters important to me can only come about if I ask for more help in the home, so I have done this.'

Others get real satisfaction out of caring for a family, and in fact this caring role is often the most important part of our self-identity rather than our disability. Alice writes: 'I don't regard myself as a "mother in a wheelchair" but as a mother of two children.' As such she shares the problems and joys common to all mothers, tiredness being her biggest difficulty.

For someone with a high level of paralysis, running a home is possible if the help is available; other people can be your 'arms and legs', as Samantha found. She is paralysed from the neck down and cannot move her hands at all. Her sons were 6 and 9 years old at the time of her accident and her husband left her a year later. With the support of Community Service Volunteers (who provide 24-hour care) she is able to run her home and gets a great deal of satisfaction from having brought up her two sons. 'I feel very proud of the way I have overcome the obstacles that have come across my path during the last nine years. I can look at my two sons who are now 18 and 15 years old and feel proud in how they have grown up.'

An environment which has been adapted to suit our needs enables many of us to be independent in our day-to-day lives. The importance of this enabling resource is highlighted when we have to spend time away from home. Molly writes, 'With practice, I can manage the bath alone and the loo – at home – but when we go on holiday, as we just did, to France for three weeks, and facilities are inconvenient or, often, non-existent, I have to rely on my husband almost totally for getting on to a "travelling pot", helping me in the bathroom, etc. I feel diminished as a person and it almost ruined our holiday.'

The tasks of daily living will usually involve much more expense after injury than they did before we were paralysed. Sometimes the cost is obvious, as when we have to pay someone to do the housework or provide personal care. But there are also more hidden costs, as Beth identifies. 'It is difficult to ascertain the exact extra costs of disability,' she writes, 'because they are often masked. I tend to have long phone calls with friends to overcome the difficulty of getting out and seeing people. Life in general is more expensive because many economy measures are not possible – like walking or using a bicycle, going to cheap hotels if travelling, etc. Clothes also get ruined by calipers and incontinence very quickly. There are also the costs of presents to people who help with shopping, gardening, etc. which I would do myself if able; long-term parking at airports because I can't get myself there by public transport; DIY jobs about the house which I would normally do myself.'

Advice and support

'I don't need pity but I could do with some help.' Violet spoke for many when she wrote this about her experience of the range of statutory services and benefits. The majority of us got very little help and many of us encountered problems with the professionals (social workers, occupational therapists, GPs, Disablement Resettlement Officers, etc.) with whom we came into contact.

We have a need for advice and support not only when we are in hospital immediately after injury but also over the years of disability, for our needs change. The inadequacies in the services available seem to arise from two fundamental problems. First, there is no one person who can co-ordinate a response to all our practical problems (housing, money, aids and equipment, personal care, etc.); instead there are a diverse number of services which seem to be in different places and with little interaction or communication with each other. If there was one person responsible for co-ordinating these different services our lives would be made a lot easier. Secondly, the medical and social services professionals, with whom we have contact once we have left hospital, often have little specialist knowledge of our situation. Indeed, by the time we return home, we are more expert in dealing with paralysis and its implications than most of the professionals working within the community, and this can give rise to difficulties in our relationships with these people.

Annie writes of her experience. 'None of the local statutory services were of much help as they knew very little of my condition and I had to advise them. Usually they were willing to help, although what they could offer was not suitable. There have been many disagreements due to lack of communication such as them deciding what I should have or do, against my better judgement. The OT and district nurses were against my moving into my own flat [she was living with her mother] and I spent many months trying to prove that it was possible. I realised from very early on that I would have to "go it alone" and became aware of my own needs and how to achieve them.' The struggle for independence for many of us (particularly for young, single tetraplegics such as Annie) has been made harder by professionals' lack of knowledge about the possibilities of independent living.

Ranjan has had a long experience of statutory services. She writes: 'In general I would say that all those services are filled with people who seem to be insensitive and ignorant of the real needs of people with spinal injuries. They lack the knowledge to help us in practical ways. I would add, however, that the awareness is getting better.' Like many of us she found that it took a long time to find out what state benefits she was entitled to, and that the most important source of information about these was other disabled people.

Other common sources of such vital information are listening to the radio and reading the newspapers. As such, it is very much a hit and miss affair as to whether we find out what we are entitled to. Sandra found out about benefits from another disabled person. 'It took two to three years to find out all I was entitled to and we only found out about rate relief two years ago – eight years after my disablement!'

Some of us have found individual professionals to be helpful and sympathetic. Lynne wrote that her GP 'was very caring and, because he didn't know much about spinal injuries, he went on a three-day course when he heard about my accident! However,' she went on, 'although the occupational therapist, social workers, district nurses gave some advice on aids, benefits, etc. they only revealed the tip of the iceberg. My education concerning aids and benefits was completed only through hard grafted research on my mother's part, my part to a certain extent, and advice from the SIA and SIA members.' Many of us owe our benefits to advice given by welfare rights or disability organisations (in other words, by voluntary organisations rather than statutory services). However, the commonest source of advice – for more than one in four of us – has been other disabled people.

A few of us have found the statutory services to be helpful. Bearing in mind the criticism of spinal units voiced in Chapter 3, it is perhaps only fair to quote Erica's praise of her spinal unit's advice and support. 'Both the medical team and the social worker were excellent. Not only did they draw my attention to the various disability pensions, etc. but they actively helped by a home visit to assess any difficulties. The consultant fought long and hard with an ALAC centre for me to have a wheelchair other than that on the DHSS list – and won.'

Lorna has been lucky in that not only did her local social services department respond to her initial needs when she left hospital but it has also responded to her changing needs. At first, alterations were made to her bungalow and a split-level cooker provided; later, major alterations were made when an electric hoist was installed.

Sometimes, the pressures under which people in the health and social services are working limit the help which they can give us. Anita wrote that her social worker was supportive 'but she acknowledged to me that she was frustrated because she could not give the help she would have liked and this was because her allocation was so great. She was under a lot of stress which she admitted and felt inadequate emotionally because she was a caring person.'

Esme has found that, owing to pressure of their work load, the service she receives from the district nurses has deteriorated over the years. 'I feel that the caring has gone and it is more a case of attending to one as quickly as possible.'

The professional who is very rarely mentioned by any of us is the Disablement Resettlement Officer (DRO), whose role is to advise and support a start or return to work following disability. It may be the case that, as women, we were often not referred to the DRO as our role as waged workers was not taken seriously. This was certainly Isabel's experience. Injured when she was 18, she writes, 'Career advice would have been wonderful – my ideas of retraining were brushed aside by doctors; they simply insisted I return home for my parents to cope with in a small mining town where job opportunities were nil.'

Becoming disabled makes life more expensive and, at the same time, threatens our ability to earn our living. Advice about waged work and assistance in getting it is therefore vitally important. Unfortunately, only 27 women who filled in our questionnaire had had any contact with the DRO, and 20 of these were dissatisfied with the service.

A number of us found that, because personal care, appropriate housing and aids and equipment were not avaliable, our spouses had to give up work to care for us. Some relied on mothers to provide this care, and sometimes this had meant that they, too, had had to give up work. Disability increases the likelihood of dependence on state benefits and on statutory services. We thus become very vulnerable to changes in the benefit system and to the services available. Our fears in the current climate are voiced by Anita when she details some of the services on which she relies. 'Incontinence aids – at the moment I can still get these on prescriptions but as more equipment gets privatised I am getting very worried. Physiotherapist – if I need a physio we have a community one, but she looks as if she is going to be another cutback soon. Care – I pay my helpers £2 an hour. This costs me a minimum of £28 per week. I rely on state benefits to do this. Gas and electric cost more as I have to keep very warm. I go into hypothermia very quickly.' She concludes, 'It is expensive to be disabled.'

Conclusion

Generally, are our daily lives very different to those of other women? The answer is that for some disability has meant a very restricted life, while for others their lives have changed very little. Our experiences depend not so much on the level of disability but on the circumstances at the time of our injury and the resources available afterwards. Independent living can only be achieved if the housing, aids, transport and personal care are there to make it possible. For those lucky enough to obtain compensation, increased purchasing power makes independence possible. However, the majority of us do not receive compensation and therefore usually have to rely on either our own earnings, those of our families, or on state benefits and local services. In most cases, the availability of advice and support from statutory agencies is vital for a return to independence.

4.

Images

Physical appearance

In Western society great emphasis is placed on 'desirable' physical appearance, and how we look is important to both women and men. The problem for us is that we do not fulfil the image of the 'body beautiful'.

One of the hardest parts of becoming disabled is acceptance of, and living with, a changed body image. Our body shape and the aids we use (a wheelchair or crutches) are the visible signs of disability. Appearance plays a very important part in interaction with other people. What is more, women face an additional problem in that our physical attractiveness is generally the way our femininity and sexuality are measured by other people.

Spinal injury changes our physical appearance and some of us find this very hard, whether we are wheelchair users or walking with the aid of crutches. A wheelchair places us at 'navel level rather than eye level,' as Martha put it. Rosalind's friend commented, without meaning to be rude, 'You've become short and fat', a disconcerting experience for someone who had been used to being tall and slim all her adult life. Crutches also change our self-image. Those who are able to walk with crutches often said they felt ungainly and awkward.

A lot of the painful emotions experienced in the months after injury are related to our changed body image. We have to get used to a different body. Samantha wrote 'I cried the first time I was given a bath and saw my skinny body. I had lost more than two stone in weight.'

Katherine hated her body in the months following paralysis and still finds it hard to accept. 'I feel a terrible shape,' she writes, 'I've muscley arms and broad shoulders, a fat stomach and twig-like legs. Yuk!'

Molly wrote 'I *hate* my tube-shaped muscle-less legs and swollen ankles; my fat abdomen and my tendency to hunch up in the wheelchair and get round-shouldered. I'm now learning how to look better by choosing clothes carefully, going swimming regularly and sitting up straight. I don't yearn after bikinis and silk stockings any more. But YES!! the body beautiful image makes me feel bitter and resentful.'

Marie says, 'I try hard to accept my body and improve on it but it's a losing battle. I'm bombarded with pictures of beautiful bodies and I just cannot compete, so I hide my flaws and try to dress as nicely as I can.'

It is not just physical appearance that we regret. Claudia, a tetraplegic in her 30s, describes how paralysis can limit interaction with other people. 'Body language from the upper chest up is limited. And limiting. Friendship gestures towards either sex, be it a hug or pouring a drink, are now clumsy and awkward – instead of natural and fluid movements.' Spasms (involuntary muscle contractions) in our paralysed limbs can also be embarrassing and add to our feeling of awkwardness.

So how do we deal with these problems of failing to live up to the physical ideals which the rest of society sets for us? Martha reacts by feeling positive about herself and insists that, although 'a chair is limiting and slows life down, my value as a human being does not diminish'.

Most of us feel better about ourselves as time goes by. Harriet, who was injured in her late teens and has since become an air traffic controller in Kenya, writes 'My changed appearance made me feel a second class person . . . I felt all was over and nobody would ever be interested in me. Over the years, this has completely changed.'

Olivia also feels positive about herself and her appearance. She was paralysed in 1983 at the age of 25. 'I have perhaps long been slightly overweight – and I never lost this, certainly not in my legs anyway, so I only had to come to

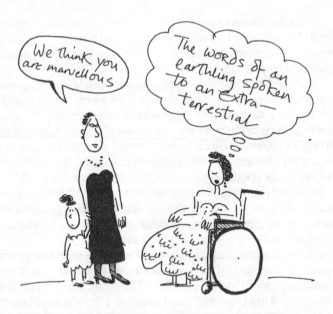

terms with my pot belly and my height!! Apart from minor periodic declines, such as sitting naked in front of a mirror, I was OK . . . When I check my appearance in front of a mirror before leaving for work I like what I see – I look and feel bright, smart and rather attractive.'

Some of us achieve these positive feelings about ourselves by valuing ourselves as people rather than for what we look like. Ingrid says that 'I have come to terms with myself as I am. I think the mind is more important than the body.' Others are like Lucy who wrote 'Now I am happy with the things I can do rather than sorry about the things I cannot do,' while some of us still value our physical appearance but stress features other than body shape.

As time passes some of us are able to be relatively philosophical about our appearance. As Liz put it, 'After all, if Bardot worried about imagined imperfections we can surely take heart from this; everyone worries about their appearance and most able-bodied women I know are more uptight about theirs than I am about mine.' Annie says, 'I have a disgusting "tetra" stomach, scars and generally feel that I look "a cripple". But I believe in the me underneath and have seen many worse looking able-bodied people, which makes me feel a little better!'

Many were concerned about putting on weight, echoing the problems faced by a lot of non-disabled women as they grow older. Most people tend to put on weight as they age, but we have the added difficulty of not being able to exercise so easily, and of extra weight being more noticeable when you are sitting down. Alison says she feels 'like a fat parcel. I am trying to lose weight for practical purposes – it's very difficult to heave oneself about when carrying too much fat.'

However, as with many features of our lives, it is difficult to separate out the effects of disability from what we would have experienced in any event. Erica, a former PE teacher, says that now she is overweight and a long way away from the athletic person she used to be. She admits, however, that although she dislikes how she looks, she thinks that sometimes she uses her disability 'as an excuse as well as a reason for not looking my best'.

Mavis points out that 'most women lose their "attractive" body shape as they age and we are not exempt'. However, Sarah does think that disability makes a difference to growing older – but this does not actually bother her that much. 'To begin with,' she wrote, 'I felt little different from my friends except for the fact of having to sit at all times. But as the years have passed, and my physical shape has deteriorated more than my peers I do find it frustrating that it can be a little more difficult to grow old gracefully. Said with tongue in cheek. For in reality few of us are perfect and appearance is not of primary concern for me.'

Clothes

Clothes are a practical issue, as well as a means of feeling positive about ourselves. It is interesting that while some felt that trousers were the most practical clothing, others thought that dresses and skirts were. What we choose to wear depends on our assessment of whether trousers or skirts are easier when getting in and out of a wheelchair or dealing with incontinence, and also what we feel about showing our legs.

Some of us felt that our disability dominated our choice of clothing, while others did not. Bridget spoke for many, however, when she said that 'I regret not being able to stand up because I think the clothes I wear would look good if I could stand up'. On the other hand, Frances is very positive about the way she looks. 'I have come to terms with myself now,' she writes, 'and am perfectly happy with my body. I dress the same way I always have, although maybe I wear skirts more as it is easier when going to the loo.'

Clothes can be a joy or a chore. Sometimes it is the practical aspects that are dominant in our choice. Nadine, for example, writes, 'I dress differently since my disability. Because of my large stomach, I now wear dresses to camouflage it. I would feel dreadfully self-conscious in fitted clothes and I do miss wearing fashionable clothes and jeans and T-shirts, etc. I find loose dresses much easier to get on and off and less likely to get wet if I am incontinent. I have to empty my bladder every two to three hours and if I had to pull trousers up and down it would take up so much time, I'd never have time for anything else. I have no incentive to buy new clothes as I know I cannot wear what I really like.'

Incontinence also dominates Geraldine's choice of clothing. 'The catheter and drainage bag I have control my choice of skirt, dresses and trousers because I can't have them short and tight as is the fashion today. I cannot wear boots either.' On the other hand, Pauline finds that using an indwelling catheter gives her greater freedom with clothing. 'When I was fighting for bladder control, having to wear incontinence pads, I used to wear trousers two sizes bigger to cope with the pads, hoping they wouldn't show. Now I have a catheter (strapped to the thigh) I wear what I want. I steer clear of front-buttoning clothes as they are difficult to get on.'

Marie finds that trousers are most suitable for her. 'I stick to trousers mostly because skirts are a nuisance when climbing in and out of cars and toilets. Sometimes I get frustrated because I love clothes and yearn for the freedom to choose what to wear.'

Margery takes a pragmatic attitude to choosing clothing but finds disability does not really dominate her choice. 'I find I choose clothes for the way they look when sitting – it is no good having decorations at the back which will not be seen and I avoid anything which will be uncomfortable to sit or lean on or cause pressure sores, also tight waists which are uncomfortable and cause bladder and digestion problems. I avoid nylon and synthetics for the lower half as it causes perspiration and promotes sores. Other than that I buy what I like and do not think it would be much different if I were walking.'

Cynthia writes, 'I dress as attractively as possible within the bounds of possibility as a paralysed person, e.g. I prefer one piece dresses as I hate to gape in the middle. Also stretchy material is comfortable. I do try to dress well but have to think of my disability when choosing.'

Over the years we work out a compromise between what kind of clothes we like and what is convenient for being in a wheelchair or using crutches. Rosalind says, 'I try to dress to express my personality but usually my choice of clothes is determined by what I feel comfortable in and what is practical and allows for ease of movement. It took me several years to find out what is easiest to wear, e.g. no narrow skirts, gathered or small pleats are best. Dresses with waists, to make the most of any shape I have and coats with wide sleeves.'

On the other hand, Vicky's assessment about what kind of skirts are best for sitting in a wheelchair indicates that maybe sometimes it is our body shape rather than the wheelchair itself which determines what we think looks best. 'I have to dress smartly for work and find the choice is very limited – skirts and dresses with pleats or gathers at the waist look untidy sitting down so I end up with plain tailored shapes which are hard to get hold of at the moment.' She goes on to describe how she gets round our common problems with trousers. 'I get trousers made to measure so that the back is much higher than the front and the bottom of the leg sits evenly along my shoes. I get pretty bored dressing this way.'

Laura was injured in a car accident in 1980 when she was 23 years old. 'Obviously my dress has been altered by the chair as I would be wearing mini-skirts, shorts and bathing suits in the summer. Now I try hard to cover my legs by canvas boots. I still wear dresses and luckily long ones are still "in". In the winter I wear more or less the same clothes. Although it is difficult to be too outrageous as it doesn't suit the chair . . . e.g. orange hair.'

Ranjan regrets that she cannot wear some of the clothes she prefers. 'I do dress mainly as I choose but there are some things such as a flowing sari and the more traditional Eastern clothes which need to hang in a certain way which I can't wear. This is because they don't look right when one is sitting down. Also I used to wear very soft dancing shoes and I can't do that now as my feet are dropping a lot and I need something with some support.'

Isabel, paralysed now for nearly 30 years, writes about how she feels about clothes. 'I choose the colours I like but usually dress to disguise my altered shape. I had been *very* thin before paralysis. I hide the thick waist with loose tops and I always wear slacks/jeans, occasionally a long dress. I would feel really uncomfortable with bare legs – at first I did not like my present partner to see them but now I'm not that self-conscious with her. I suspect that by dressing to hide this changed shape I may succeed in fooling myself that really I do look the same – sometimes I can even *feel* thin, though I know I'm not. I dress in what is comfortable for me – I would feel less comfortable in skirts and close-fitting clothes.'

Disability has converted at least one of us to the advantages of English summers. Molly writes, 'If I can hide my legs under long skirts, trousers or high boots, I do – and feel a lot more confident because nobody can see them. Summer is *agony* because I have to expose more of myself than I'd like in order to be comfortably cool (thank God we live in England!)'

Wearing calipers and using crutches can bring their own problems as far as clothes are concerned. Beth says 'In the wheelchair, I can dress as I like, shoes included. But if I'm wearing calipers it is difficult to find trousers with wide enough legs, and zips have to be put in all inside seams, right up to the thigh, which is not possible with most jeans. When wearing skirts, the knee joints of the two calipers interlock and cause me to fall; also skirts show more leg. Shoes strong enough to take full length calipers are almost impossible to come by.' She goes on, 'Although these things have to be borne in mind, I don't think disability dominates my dress. I bear it in mind the way I give consideration to colouring. The mini-skirt was, however, a sore trial!'

Rachel walks with splints (wooden supports placed at the back of the legs) and has adapted her clothing style to suit them. 'I have had modern leather boots made in various colours incorporating splints designed by myself, so I can continue to dress as fashionably as my purse will allow. It also means that instead of always wearing trousers to hide my splints I can now wear skirts. I only show my splints at home or on holiday, not because they bother me so much as because people continuously ask what their purpose is.'

Christine was paralysed when she was 21 in 1958 and walks with knee calipers and a stick. She writes of her changed body image – 'I have never had much problem with this once I got over my initial dislike of calipers. I just dress the way I like *except* I have to wear trousers and boots for about eight months of the year, to keep warm. I *prefer* skirts, though.'

Shoes were a problem mentioned by many of us. Claire wrote 'The main item of clothing I have trouble with is shoes, i.e. court shoes and sandals tend to fall off; ankle boots are OK but always hard to get on. Lace up shoes seem to be the best answer.' Rachel had overcome her problems with splints by buying made-to-measure boots in various colours, but those of us using calipers bemoaned the limitations of finding shoes strong enough to fit the calipers to. Rosalind voices a common frustration when she writes, 'I find it very traumatic buying shoes and long to wear elegant high heels!'

When clothing becomes, or remains, a joy for us, it is often because we emphasise colours and style. Bridget finds that she dresses in brighter colours than she used to. She takes pleasure in co-ordinating colours, particularly in choosing long dangling earrings to go with the clothes she is wearing. Tessa says 'I wear maternity style dresses quite a lot but they have to look nice to be acceptable and in fact they look much better on a sitting person than on a standing one, anyway.'

Dreams

We put a question about dreams in the questionnaire because it is fascinating to know what our subconscious is up to when we're asleep. Interestingly, very few of us dream of ourselves as disabled. The majority never see ourselves as disabled in our dreams, while some said that this aspect of ourselves varied. It is intriguing that most of us have similar dreams in which we experience an ability to walk, but also some difficulty with walking.

Of those who never dream of being disabled, many saw themselves as being very active. Phyllis said: 'I often dream I am running free through beautiful fields.' Molly dreams of running or dancing, while Liz dreams of 'flying or floating'. Beryl writes: 'Thank goodness I never dream that I am disabled but always walking or running. It is wonderful to go to sleep.' While in hospital Olivia often dreamed of being a marathon runner, but she did not think this was a pleasant experience. As she said, 'it was not the best way to start a new day.'

The most common type of dream is that in which we can walk almost normally but are hindered in some way. This was described by Melanie who wrote 'I'm never in a wheelchair but I always have very heavy legs which I'm either dragging or can't lift', and Martha who said 'sometimes I'm aware I'm disabled but I'm walking – other times I'm in my chair but using my legs – to brake or push. A few times I realise I can move them after all – I just haven't tried hard enough.' A former dancer, Gina, wrote that she sometimes dreams she was a 'bit shaky' on her legs and needed 'to do some exercises'.

Wheelchairs often figure in dreams, as Claire describes. 'I can usually walk in my dreams but the dreaded chair is always lurking around somewhere.' Her most frequent dream is one in which she can stand up and walk about, but as soon as she sits down she is paralysed again! Annie wrote that she never saw herself in a wheelchair but sometimes she sees a wheelchair not belonging to her 'with no one in it'.

Mavis is one of the few of us who is always disabled in her dreams. Now bedfast, she writes, 'I am always disabled and always trying to get out of some awkward situation e.g. locked in a large rambling building and unable to reach a door or window to call for help. This has been worse since I found a burglar by my bed two years ago in the middle of the night. I think dreaming is good for me, at least when I wake I have all my aids around me and I am back to independence again.'

Several of us mentioned a preoccupation with finding toilets when dreaming! Lindy writes: 'I never dream of myself as disabled but always looking for toilets.' Carol said that she often dreamed of 'using toilets in very public places' and Tessa said that when she dreams of being disabled she can walk with two sticks (in reality she cannot) and that she has learnt that this means 'I want to go to the toilet. Why, I don't know, but I get up fast.'

Some of us wrote of dreaming of being both able-bodied and disabled in the same dream. Bronwen, who was paralysed nearly 40 years ago, said that she can suddenly change in mid-dream and described how she once dreamed that she 'carried my car above my head across a sandy beach to keep the grit out of the works!' Someone else who has amazing dreams is Celia who dreamed that she ran up a rough hillside to collect her crutches.

Aspects other than disablement are sometimes more important in influencing our dreams. Erica writes: 'like everyone else with a weight problem my dreams are usually dominated by a "slim" image of myself – not an image without a wheelchair.' Elsa, whose 7-year-old daughter was killed in the same accident which left her paralysed in 1983, is relieved that she does not dream much at the moment. 'I rarely dream now – and this I consider a blessing as I *could* have a lot to have nightmares about. I have only twice had a dream in which I was in a chair and I considered the first of these to be a breakthrough in acceptance of the disability. I have had the odd bad dream about losing my remaining child.'

Geraldine has the ultimate revenge on the non-disabled world when she dreams. She writes: 'In my dreams I am never disabled but everyone else is.'

'There's a lot of us about . . . '

How we feel about ourselves is often tied up with how we feel about disability and disabled people in general. All of us have had ambivalent feelings about other disabled people. These feelings may stem from non-disabled people lumping us all together because we supposedly have so much more in common with each other than with the non-disabled world. Frances, for example, 'hates being pushed together with other disabled people just because we are disabled. My friends from before my accident are still my friends.'

Liz, who has been a paraplegic for over 20 years, wrote that 'with other disabled people my reactions are much the same as they would be with anyone else. Either you get on and have shared interests and an innate liking, or you don't.' She values the 'place of shared experiences' but cautions against automatically expecting 'durable friendship if your disability is all you have in common'.

Helen is very resistant to the 'disabled' label and her feelings reflect the usual negative associations with the term 'disabled'. She writes 'I have very little contact with other disabled people through choice. We try to live as a normal family in an able-bodied world and I certainly don't want my children to grow up surrounded by disability. To me, the label disabled means "poor" and we're not poor, either financially or spiritually. For a long time I would not refer to myself as disabled but found it necessary to use the term to claim benefits and other forms of help.'

Frances also objects to the label. 'I hate the word disabled. I am just as able as anyone – it's just that I cannot walk. I get about and do as much as I did before. I hate being fussed over. If I want help I would rather ask for it than be asked every 10 seconds if I can manage.'

It is the impact of our disability when we are 'in public' which is often so difficult to deal with. As Sarah said, 'The concept of being labelled "disabled" to me means that it's almost impossible to merge into a crowd.' Ursula is very clear about the disadvantages that disability brings: ' "Disabled" means a group of people who are discriminated against by the majority of the public,' she says.

Barbara has conflicting feelings about the impact she makes in public. 'I used to feel apologetic, guilty. I felt like saying "I'm sorry I'm in a wheelchair and causing this upheaval" or "making you feel embarrassed". But also I could feel the very opposite – it's only by a commotion being made that able-bodied people will think of access, loos, etc. And it's only by being seen in public that wheelchair users will be accepted, and the general public become accustomed to the fact that *there's a lot of us about and more to come.*'

Lynne wrote of how her attitude towards disability has changed as a result of becoming disabled herself. 'Before my accident I had never really come across or thought about disability. I thought that anyone who broke their neck would die instantly and that people with disabilities were the brave strugglers in society. Now I am doing all I can to persuade other people that I come across that this is not so. People with disabilities are the same as able-bodied people in many important ways – we have needs, wishes, dreams, sexuality, bouts of depression, good days and bad days. We do not want to be thought of as brave heroes!'

Margery also tries to educate other people: 'I am a Women's Institute speaker on disability and speak to many other groups as well. I try to promote the idea of "people with disabilities" just as we have "people with red hair".'

We may hate being disabled but we are not necessarily overwhelmed by the restrictions on our lives. Charlotte wrote: 'My feelings are ambivalent. I hate being disabled, but accept it now as something I can't change so must make the best of a bad thing. I have learnt to live my life which is governed by being disabled, but try not to let it influence my life and what I want to do any more than I can help. I don't feel disabled, only a person who has a disability. The early things which cause frustration I have overcome and now find the frustrations of being disabled in more ambitious things I'd like to do, for example, to sail a large dinghy and race.'

The negative image of disability also makes it more difficult to be with other people with disabilities 'in public'. As Patsy put it, being with others like ourselves 'brings home to us our predicament'. The public view of disability means that Beth, for instance, admitted 'I am honestly not at ease with disabled people in public, though perfectly at ease in private, when we can relate to each other without spectators who define us as disabled'. She feels 'conspicuous and rather ridiculous when there are more than one of us out together – as if we lose our individuality and just become a group of the disabled'.

Norma echoes this: 'I feel at ease with other disabled people but I do not like it if we are all placed together at any functions as if we are a different species; it makes me more aware of my own disabilities.'

On the other hand, Mavis stresses the shared experience of people with disabilities. 'We have a common bond and understand the problems which might affect one person and not another. We uplift one another because, with luck, our "bad patches" do not always happen at the same time. We know what lack of independence and freedom of movement mean from first hand.'

Marie gets fed up with always having to be the one to make the first move in forming friendships with able-bodied people and she feels 'it's a relief to be with other disabled people where I don't have to do this or explain anything. I can relax more in their company.'

Many of us find it difficult to relate to people whose disability is unfamiliar to us, although some are also wary of what is sometimes recognised as 'the arrogance of groups of spinally injured to other disabilities' (as Karen put it). Tessa wrote: 'I am far more worried about whether an epileptic person will have a fit than by being with someone with a disability, because of the uncertain change in them and not knowing what to expect.' Similarly, Linda does not find it easy to relate to people with severe mental handicaps, and Ellen confesses to being ill at ease with people with cerebral palsy because, as she put it 'I don't want to be considered deficient' in the way that they are. Having admitted to these ambivalent and uncomfortable feelings, however, many of us, including Linda and Ellen, are trying hard to overcome our own negative attitudes as we suffer so much from such attitudes ourselves.

Isabel has found that very positive things have come from her involvement with disability issues. 'I seem to become more and more positive about my disability and can't avoid seeing it positively now. "Disabled" to me means a physical or mental impairment but it doesn't mean unnatural or useless. Sometimes, though, I think I have had it easy, being only paraplegic and not tetraplegic. If you have the use of hands, eyes and brain, and little pain, you've got a good start. Disability hasn't stopped me doing most of the things I enjoy e.g. reading, writing, watching nature, sky, stars, sewing, artwork. Getting to know more and more disabled people has been, and is, a joy. There's a special strength and solidarity about it, even more than I have found in the lesbian/ gay community. It's like finding kinship for the first time. I used years ago to have resistance to being "with my own kind" but this was because it was being thrust on me. To *choose* to be with other disabled people, to share and work with them, is a liberation. I only wish this had happened sooner. Joining with the first other disabled lesbian I met to form a national network has been especially rewarding.'

'Does she take sugar? . . .'

Other people's attitudes and comments can often make us feel disabled in a way that the disability itself does not. Most of us, on a daily and continuing basis, are reminded that we are seen as different and it is this loss of anonymity in a crowd that we regret so keenly.

Strangers in the street have a range of responses to us, from the 'How marvellous you are!' through ignorance to very obvious fear of the alien nature of disability. Our common experience is that it is unlikely that we can go out in public, to the shops, the theatre, the library, to pick our children up from school, etc., without encountering some reaction from a total stranger. Libby says, 'Some days I get really angry at the way people stare at me in the street. I feel like saying "I don't have three heads, do I?" but most of the time I accept it – after all I stare at disabled people myself. I am nearly always very self-conscious in public; I don't like being in situations which attract too much attention. I hate it when mothers grab their toddlers out of the way, saying "Mind the lady, darling", even though I know they're only trying to be considerate.'

Tessa wrote: 'I have an "automatic smile" which tends to pop out when people say silly things regardless of what I feel inside. I still find myself wondering what to say to total strangers who ask why I'm in a chair.' But what *do* we feel inside?

Our experiences and reactions vary, but very few of us express what we feel as a result of other people's remarks. As Patsy says, 'Naturally, I could punch them straight in the face when they're patronising – but one has to bite one's tongue, smile and put it down to ignorance.' Laura also hides her feelings: 'Sometimes I feel aggressive inside about the comments but never say anything rude.'

Many of us fume inside, like Beryl, who writes, 'I cannot stand people whom I have never met smiling, like cheshire cats, at me in my chair or the attitude adopted by someone, for example, who recently said "We think you are so patient". This makes me feel like exploding!! The "Does she take sugar?" attitude, or someone answering questions on my behalf – I cannot describe the fury it generates.'

Some encounters are very upsetting. Pauline wrote: 'Many people are patronising and condescending . . . the worst comment I get is "What a shame, you're so pretty" – only because I try to make the best of myself. The obvious reply is "Would you feel better if I was an ugly frump?" '

Phyllis wrote of her range of reactions to different types of people: 'I cope with the ignorant by joking and trying to laugh away their discomfort. If rude pointed remarks are passed I go conveniently deaf. If people are genuinely concerned I discuss the matter with them briefly and to the point. I do not think I'm marvellous and I tell them so.'

Many of us get the 'I do think you're marvellous!' reaction. This can provoke complex feelings. As Leila wrote, 'I just say I was lucky, which I was. To explain my motives for survival, or at some stages my lack of need to survive, would involve too much self-explanation. I don't get close enough to people to want them to know me that well. So I just smile but inside ignore what they're saying.' Georgina stressed: 'I do hate the expression about "being marvellous" as I just get on with life in the best possible way.'

However positive we feel about ourselves and how we are coping, other people's remarks about how marvellous we are can be difficult to deal with. This is because the unspoken comment is that it's a miracle that we manage at all. 'It strains one's patience!' said Elspeth. 'Yes, we know how marvellous we are to face the world with what appears to be serenity and cheerfulness, and we refrain from saying how little idea, in truth, they have.'

Eileen writes: 'I agree with anyone who thinks I'm marvellous – it's easier than denying it. The ones who tell me how brave I am usually shut up when I ask them what alternative I've got.' On the other hand, Pamela remarks, 'I tend to lose my cool if people tell me how brave I am, since I do not regard learning to live reasonably successfully with a disability as a particularly courageous action.'

Whatever our feelings about how well we 'cope' with our disability, and why, it's clear that the 'how marvellous you are!' remarks are rarely a sincere valuation of our worth but more often patronising comments on how awful it must be to be disabled. This is very difficult to cope with when, as Yvonne wrote, 'I feel – this is me. I'm not marvellous. I'm

living my life as normally as possible and I want as few concessions as possible.'

Olivia has some suggestions for retorts to inane remarks:
'Don't be so pathetic!'; 'I may be pushing myself around but
at least I'm not carrying dead weight on top of my shoulders'; and 'I may be paralysed from the waist downwards
but I'm not dead from the neck upwards'. However, many
of us have concluded, particularly after some years of living
with our 'differentness', that we have to adopt a 'smile and
ignore them' policy. It's the least complicated approach
when we have neither the time nor the inclination to chal-
lenge glib and sometimes hurtful remarks.

Harriet demonstrates how careful we sometimes are when
in public. 'I am always ready for stares,' she writes, 'looks of
pity and lots of sympathy – but all this tells me how much
"help" these people need from me. I make sure I never look
gloomy or sad. A smile is the best tonic to the public. Show
them you are happy and do not give a damn about their
looks. In the case of comments, I always try to give a positive rather than a negative response – or else they'll think
you are defeated and are complaining if you make the mistake of being rude.'

Some of us have become impervious (almost) to other
people's reactions. As Edith remarked, 'I've long ceased to
care about what anyone thinks of me – though I do hate to
look awkward and clumsy which I fear I often do.' Angela's
confidence in herself helps her to deal with other people. 'I
treat everyone equally. Being patronised does not irritate
me any more. I do know my own worth.' She finds that it is
her friends who continue to be irritated by other people's
patronising reactions to her.

Many of us have tried to understand why people react in
the way that they do. 'People do not understand until it has
happened to them, and no amount of literature, lectures and
so on is going to change that. Unfortunately, only personal
experience will.' Therefore, Julia concluded, 'retorting with
a sarcastic comment is not, in my mind, the answer.'

Alix agrees. 'I find it pointless getting steamed up as
usually it's "well meant". Ugh! Sometimes I put them right

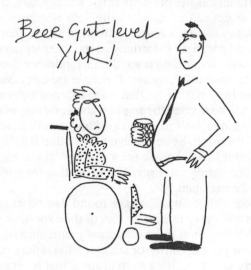

Beer Gut level
YuK!

but not aggressively as that tends to be counterproductive.'
Nadine tries to understand why people behave in the way
they do. 'I try to treat them and talk to them as normally as I
can,' she says, 'and hope that they will soon forget about my
wheelchair. I am probably the only wheelchair person they
know and they are unsure of how to treat me. They don't
realise how many other people say "Have you passed your
test yet?" so you have to try to smile sweetly and act as if it's
the first time you've heard it.'

Wendy is charitable. 'Overall, most people don't realise
they're being patronising and I try to think how I reacted to
disabled people before the accident.' And more than one of
us admitted that before our own disability we would walk
on the other side of the street rather than be confronted by
that kind of reality. Karen wrote: 'Why blame people for
their reactions? Is it their fault that they don't understand
my situation? A lot of the time ı can see the funny side.'

We all have to deal with unsolicited offers of help when
we go out in public, and when we do not need help this can

cause difficulty as people quite often will not take no for an answer, or get offended when the help is refused. In this situation, Linda says 'I find it difficult to accept help gracefully when I could do something so much easier myself'.

As Blanche says, 'Help is so often a hindrance if one cannot give precise instructions.' If people are offended when we refuse help it may be that they will not offer it again when it may be needed (by us or by someone else with a disability). We are therefore put in a difficult position. Madeline writes: 'I try not to be aggressive when offered help I don't want – and if I *really* don't want it, I say "No thanks, I can manage but thank you for offering" so that they won't be put off offering again.'

It is clear that most of us have found that other people's reactions are a very important part of the experience of disability. It's almost as if our disability grants unwritten permission for people to pry or stare or offer solutions when none were asked for. It's a form of stress that is very seldom recognised. Each intrusion proves yet again that we are seen as different and separate and no longer part of the general stream of life. 'I hate being different,' says Violet – but is it the disability which makes her different or the change in people's attitudes and reactions towards her?

Our feelings about other people's attitudes can be summed up by Marie who wrote, 'People need to be educated. I find it hard to cope, though, with ignorance, pity and the "Does s/he take sugar?" syndrome. I can cope with my problems, but people are sometimes difficult. It's people and the environment that make life in a wheelchair hard.'

Many of us react with anger and upset, even after years in a wheelchair; all of us try to understand and come to terms with this aspect of our disability. Liz concludes: 'I feel it is vital to accept that no one is going to see you as you really are to yourself and not to fight their prejudice. They don't know that they are being patronising and cruel. We, too, are probably guilty of the same prejudices to other minorities – what is different is always persecuted.'

Conclusion

Has our disability fundamentally affected our self-image? Just less than half of us felt that it had, while over half felt that it had not. Magda spoke for many when she wrote, 'I am still me except that my legs don't work' and Bronwen, who has been disabled for over 25 years, said, 'I don't feel that I have changed a great deal. I think I have more patience and a greater understanding of others, but perhaps this would have happened with advancing years anyway.'

Some of us feel that we are basically the same but that some characteristics of ourselves have become intensified. Linda, a solicitor in her 40s, said she felt 'more aggressive, more determined, because the obstacles are so much greater'.

We all experience an initial feeling of loss when newly injured. For some the grief persists. Libby, an incomplete tetraplegic who walks with sticks, wrote, ' "Disabled" means to me being weaker and more defenceless, being unpleasantly different. I was a person who very much enjoyed physical activity and now I feel as if a large and important part of the person I was no longer exists. After seven years I still haven't come to terms with this absence, like a sudden death.'

Annie writes about how she feels about being disabled. 'I usually try not to think too deeply about it. I have to divide the meaning of "happiness" to say I am now happy with whatever but not with being disabled. Being disabled is so against my every instinct that I *still* go to "get up" when the phone rings! I suffer too much emotional conflict to come properly to terms with the situation, though despite this I incredibly seem to have survived and even more incredibly can still experience great joy and happiness. Generally I feel good about myself and would not wish to be anyone else.'

5.

Sexuality and Relationships

The public image of someone with a disability is of a person alone, often elderly. Although it is estimated that one in four families in Britain contains someone with a learning or physical disability, there is very little knowledge about how disability affects relationships, how it affects someone's role as a lover, for example.

Disability brings about many changes and our sexuality is an important part of ourselves which is affected. As in all areas of our lives, the effect on our sexual relationships and how we feel about ourselves apropos of sex, depends to a large extent on the circumstances before our injury. However, the constraints of our social identity as 'disabled' also have a profound effect on our sexuality.

Overnight we pass into a state where many people assume we are asexual, often in order to hide embarrassment about the seemingly incongruous idea that such 'abnormal' people can have 'normal' feelings and relationships. As Anita wrote, 'on the whole I think society wishes to view us as asexual because to think differently challenges many of its own prejudices about sex and the disabled. I mean – should we actually be allowed it?'

Pauline also gives voice to this experience. 'I was made to feel "crude" or labelled sex-mad because I wanted to resume a normal life. It appeared that, once disabled, it was wrong to think of sexuality – disabled people didn't do that sort of thing!'

Young women in particular can find their families consider them to be asexual. Liz, who was ill for a year following her climbing accident when she was 18, wrote, 'Once I'd recovered enough to look good again I felt I was sexually attractive but kept it quiet. Family and friends treated me as a write-off in that area. They so affected my self-respect in this that when men were attentive I thought they were just being kind. They had to be quite insistent before I dared believe they wanted me.' When she finally embarked on a sexual relationship, she felt 'delight, elation, triumph at the vindication of instinct over conditioning. Anger that I'd ever been duped into betraying my instinct by the attitudes that had written me off as an incomplete woman, or that sex was only possible in the text-book manner.'

On the other hand, those of us who are happy without a sexual relationship can be made to feel deprived or incomplete because of this. The assumption is often made that, if we do not have a partner, our single state must be something which has been forced upon us rather than positively chosen. Such social pressures make it difficult for women who do not have sexual relationships to view their lives positively. Social pressures also make it more difficult for lesbians to speak openly about their relationships. Unfortunately, this has meant that our questionnaires contained very little material about lesbian relationships or positive accounts of celibacy. There is therefore a regrettable, but unavoidable, failure in this chapter to fully represent either of these two experiences.

Body image and sexuality

We have to deal with our feelings about our bodies and whether or not we still feel the same about our sexuality after our injuries.

We had varying reactions to changes in our physical shape and how we felt it affected our sexuality. Did we feel less sexually attractive after paralysis? Almost all of us answered yes to this question, but the intensity of our feelings varied.

Catrin wrote about how she felt 'like a woman with

anorexia and didn't like to show my legs or backside. I wasted away quite considerably in my bottom half and am very conscious of it.' She now feels a lot more positive about herself and comments, 'Yes, there are some men in the world that just aren't attracted to paraplegic women, but in actual fact they have the problem – themselves.' She advises: 'Your partner accepts your body in time but make sure you tell him about things. If he doesn't accept you he's a jerk and is not right for you – it's as easy as that.' She admits, however, that sometimes she is affected by the 'body beautiful' image. 'I'm very women's lib minded and it makes me sick how women's bodies are exploited all the time. My downfall is down at the beach with my partner – and all those beautiful brown figured bodies in swimsuits.'

Erica finds it impossible to feel at ease with her changed body. 'At the time of leaving hospital', she wrote, 'I looked very drawn, thin and grey-faced.' She still feels unattractive, although now for different reasons. 'I have gained almost three stone in weight which leaves me two stone overweight and it shows. I still try to cover myself during making love as I hate my fat body. I have tried to lose weight but deep down feel it wouldn't alter my own image of my present self.'

Although many of us found that we lost our sexual identity when we were first disabled, as time went on most started to feel more positive about ourselves. This was the experience of Geraldine, who wrote, 'I did feel less sexually attractive, because I was surrounded by metal and wheels, and had no control over my body, bladder and bowels. I needed help with everything and couldn't possibly see how men could find me sexually attractive.' Her views have since 'totally changed'. Although she thought no one would ever want to make love to her, her experiences of relationships, and now marriage, have proved her wrong.

Isabel, paralysed 28 years ago when she was 18, continues to be critical of her body shape. But, she says, 'I am more conscious most people are fairly ordinary and don't have beautiful bodies. I still feel surprise, though, when someone other than my present mate says that she fancies me.'

Olivia is one of the few women who found that she did not feel less sexually attractive immediately following her paralysis. She did feel 'shy and unsure of my body and its responses – but not bashful and not afraid of speaking my mind (as long as the lights were out!!). As time passes,' she continues, 'and experience of being in a chair increases, confidence grows tremendously and my personality shines out and I feel very, very attractive, taking great care of my appearance.'

Happy ever after?

Many of us – whether lesbians or heterosexual – have found that our partners at the time of our disability still love us; if we did not have a sexual relationship at the time, that we have since formed lasting relationships. However, like couples in the non-disabled world, many have also experienced divorce and difficult relationships.

Sixty-six women were single at the time of injury and 46 remained so, some because they choose to and are happy with their single state, and some with regret. Sometimes the shock of disablement breaks up a relationship, but just as often it seems to bring people closer together. Our disability is an added dimension in our relationships with other people rather than the only determining characteristic.

One hundred and two women were married or cohabiting at the time of injury. Of these, 73 were in the same relationship at the time of filling in the questionnaire and 12 had been widowed (some in the same accident which caused the disability). Seventeen marriages ended in divorce in the years following paralysis.

Samantha blames her divorce partly on her consultant who told her husband that '75 per cent of marriages go bang and to get rid of our double bed. I am sure this stayed with him and did not give our personal life a chance. He left 15 months after I came home.'

Theresa was a 35-year-old mother of three young sons when she became a tetraplegic as a result of a car accident.

Her marriage ended in divorce soon afterwards and she writes of her husband 'He was not the type to accept disability. As far as he was concerned I was only "half a woman"!'

The very sudden change in our circumstances usually places an existing relationship under a lot of strain. Erica wrote: 'Any changes in our relationship were caused by frustrations. I was very aware that my husband wasn't sure how to react to me in all sorts of situations, from making love to household chores. My determination to be independent made me spurn help at first and then, as I invariably did too much, we argued. It's almost three years now since I came home and even now we are still unsure of each other at times.'

Marion, who was injured in 1983, is concerned about the obstacles that her disability poses to her sexual relationship with her husband. 'I knew how important our sex life was during our 28 years of married life. It was the first thing I asked the doctors about. As I have to use a catheter it has put my husband off our normal love making. My spasms [involuntary muscle contractions] are so strong that normal sex is impossible. I think my husband is still in shock. He is also 59 years old but this does not mean we have given up. It is early days and we love each other dearly. I hope that in the future we can experiment with other ways. We used to share a double bed but now we sleep separately. This has a lot to do with our love life but there is no way yet that we can share a bed.'

Molly, who gradually became more paralysed over a number of years as a result of a spinal tumour, writes of the adjustments that occurred within her relationship. 'It was strained sometimes because I found things physically difficult to do and was tired/irritable/frustrated lots of the time. I felt inadequate as a partner and was convinced my husband didn't want to be seen with me and that I should be playing squash with him or going mountain-climbing. I also felt sexually inadequate and was *convinced* every other woman he met was more attractive than I was. Things have changed now. I am more self-confident. I've sussed out how to do things around the house with relative ease. The children are older and don't need watching/carrying/cleaning every other minute. I also have a social life of my own as well as the one we have together. I'm happier and that rubs off. We had a period of almost separating six years ago and it jolted us so much we both took stock and realised what we had was basically good. It's improved since.'

Sometimes a relationship does not survive the tremendous strains placed on it by disability. Marie became engaged to her boyfriend following her motor bike accident when she was 16, but writes 'it didn't last because he kept wrapping me in cotton wool which at first I needed. But then I had to learn how to live again and he wouldn't let me go. I wanted to go to college but he didn't want me to. So I went anyway and that finished it.'

Some of us find that a relationship with a man is under added strain following our disability because our roles as women are so bound up with caring for a male partner. Some men find it very difficult to take on the caring role, and this was certainly why Julia felt her marriage broke up. 'Paralysis destroyed this marriage,' she wrote. 'The facts were he could not stand the thought of looking after a disabled woman or the thought of sex with me, so he quickly found someone else.' And Louise wrote: 'Our marriage has really stopped existing. If my husband did not have to be so much of my carer, especially of a personal nature, things might be easier.'

Yvonne also wrote that, although her sexual relationship with her husband has improved since her paralysis, they row a lot because 'my husband has found the strain of supporting me, running the home and family initially and keeping the business going very hard.' She fears that he 'sometimes feels tied to a cripple which limits our social life. He enjoyed having an attractive wife and the competitive element, "You can look but she chose me" is not quite so applicable'.

Pamela writes of how her relationship has changed since her car accident in 1972. 'My disability decreased my confidence in myself; it made me desperately apologetic and anxious to please. My husband, because I have to rely on him so much (e.g. shopping), has become increasingly auto-cratic. He resents any expression of an opinion contrary to his own. He always needs to be right, to be in control. The relationship has adapted by the submerging (by me) of my right to my own opinion and the acceptance of my hus-band's. I would rather lose my self-respect than lose him. On major points of difference I will express my views, but ultimately I will always accept his (with mental reservations, none the less!). This isn't necessarily a consequence of my disability, however – our relationship was veering in this direction anyway and my disability accelerated and empha-sised existing trends rather than initiating new ones.'

On the other hand, some of us found that our partners responded in a supportive and helpful way, and in some instances the relationship improved. Fiona found that her disability has brought her closer to her husband. As the breadwinner in her household, she had been more outgoing and involved in things outside the home than her husband. 'We are probably more bound together now. We have joked?? that my disability is our shared interest and hobby. I did a lot on my own before paralysis, and we may have reached a stage where we were drifting dangerously apart. My spouse is a home bird. I am now more of a home bird. He has been astonishingly supportive but treats me as "nor-mal". There have been a lot of changes anyway in the last four years. The children have left home. My mother-in-law has moved in. My husband has become more sociable and outgoing generally. I have valued him even more.'

Mavis writes of how her husband reacted to her initial paralysis 22 years ago as the result of a spinal tumour. She became confined to her bed 10 years ago and when her hus-band retired four years later he took over all the personal care that she needs. She writes: 'Our feelings of love for one another have grown over our 31 years of marriage and are still growing. We cannot imagine life without one another in spite of the fact that we are not sexually active. We feel that our love for one another has not been impaired by my dis-ability.'

Both Fiona and Mavis are writing of relationships which

were already well established at the time of their disability. However, some relationships which were very new also survived the strain. Kathy was paralysed in the early days of her relationship. In 1979 she developed a spinal abscess just four weeks after her marriage to a man whom she had met only 16 weeks before. Her initial reaction was that she was no longer sexually attractive because she could not dress 'in sexy clothes (i.e. mini-skirts, tight jeans). Also I couldn't wriggle my bum anymore.' She was at first very frightened of making love, but now writes, 'My husband and I both enjoy a very active sex life. He makes me feel normal. My husband made me strong. I think if it wasn't for him I would have given up but now – I am a fighter. We love and enjoy each other very much.'

Isabel, who formed her (lesbian) relationship with her partner six years after her disability, although they had known each other for longer, writes that although 'disability is irksome in that there are some things we'll never do together, there are so many other things we share – leisure activities as well as voluntary and campaigning work. We become closer all the time and the years together seem to go by all too quickly.'

Olivia writes of the impact of her injury on her relationship. 'It had the effect of making me aware that my partner loved me, the basic inside personality me, and not the 5′ 7″ brunette walker. He visited me in hospital every day; being together gave us ample opportunity to discuss everything many many times over. One other factor is that he works away from home for periods of between three to five months. Letters are our main communication and they arrived six at a time and none for two to three weeks. Through long, longing letters, our love grew and grew and my confidence soared. Some factors in the "normal" day-to-day relations are never mentioned and perhaps forgotten or taken for granted, but letters give a deeper insight into each other and yourself, a medium for expressing inner feelings, beliefs and desires. They are brought into the foremind, written down and exchanged. Brimming full of love and confidence leads to a brighter bubbly person – well it did in me. Our relationship has strengthened over the few years since the accident. We've recently married and are very very happy.'

Karen stresses that it is important not to blame disability for everything – 'You must not put down to paralysis the normal strains of marriage'. Isabel is aware of this tendency, saying 'if we parted I would probably relate it to the disability though my rational mind knows this is not necessarily so.'

Isabel also writes about how her disablement initially made her eager to prove herself by rushing into a relationship. Bridget echoes this in her account of her attitude towards her relationship with her child's father. She writes: 'I had finished my relationship with my child's father while I was pregnant. I am (and was) very happy living on my own with her. However, immediately after my accident I tried to make my relationship with her father work again. Partly this was because of the pressure to at least provide my daughter with a "normal" nuclear family. This was a mistake and didn't last for very long. It wasn't my disability which prevented it from working but rather all the problems that were there anyway. I thought that somehow my disability would make it work because I needed him. In fact, I didn't need him and the relationship was over, anyway.'

Orgasms

Most of us, following paralysis, cannot experience orgasms in the same way that we did before. This is either because we have only incomplete feeling in vagina and clitoris or because we have no sensation at all. We have many different feelings about this and ways of dealing with it.

Those of us who have incomplete sensation often find that it takes a long time before we can experience an orgasm again. Pamela was very concerned about whether she would ever be able to reach orgasm again 'and nobody seemed to know (or even be very concerned, apart from my husband!) My early doubts and anxieties hampered my sexual response until about 18 months after the birth of my son, when I had been seeing an obstetrician and gynaecologist. He made various practical suggestions about ways to increase the intensity of my response and finally I discovered I could still climax – although the sensation was somewhat different from my memories. This mattered to me enormously and tremendously increased my self-confidence – I no longer felt such a failure!'

Catrin writes of the importance of taking time when making love. 'After the first few times I had sex, I still could not get as much pleasure as my partner was getting from me. I felt I was able to satisfy him but found it difficult to get full pleasure unless foreplay was prolonged.' Karen says that it took years before she had an orgasm again. 'I now know more about the right position. My husband finds it difficult to believe that I cannot physically feel intercourse. He says it's just the same as before.'

Some of us who have no sensation in our vaginas or clitorises find that we can experience equivalent orgasms through sensations in other parts of our bodies. Beth, injured when she was 14, writes 'gradually I found that though without vaginal or clitoral sensation, other erogenous zones compensate and that if the relationship is good it is possible to reach orgasm.'

Tessa describes the joy that she finds in her sexual relationship. 'We get a great deal of pleasure from the sex I can manage. I am fairly sure I get what are called "phantom orgasms" and we are always game to try new experiments and positions. It is definitely true to say that we get far more enjoyment from sex than we ever thought possible. We use mouth and nose and facial stroking a great deal, with back tickling as well. We both get thoroughly turned on by these things and we culminate by my husband entering me. I am very ticklish in certain places and I can get an orgasm from being stroked there (for example, under my arms). If most people felt as good as we do, I think they'd be very happy. Love is wonderful stuff and transcends just about everything.'

A number of us stress that orgasm is not the most important

thing about a sexual relationship. Isabel, speaking of her lesbian relationship, writes, 'There is lots of fun and enjoyment left; finding out what you like/don't like is good. If you can do so, stroke and touch your body yourself to find out and to get confidence. Confidence and pleasure in being yourself is important.'

Olivia wrote of her pleasure in her relationship. 'I would suggest to other women don't let anyone put you off. Slowly and patiently you and your partner should explore your body; know where his hands are, follow them with yours, know how he's touching you, where, and enjoy the fantastic sensations. No feeling does not equate no sensation. Explore all possible erogenous zones – breasts, neck, ears, tummy button – don't be swayed by what you read (not even in this book!). It's not how often you make love, how many times you achieve orgasm; it is enjoying your own body and your partner's! You'll only get out what you put in – in any activity. Don't ever be in a hurry and don't ever stay silent.'

Many of us, however, find it very hard to come to terms with the lack of sensation. Gina thought that difficulties with their sexual relationship contributed to her splitting up with her boyfriend. 'It's a big strain on top of all the other problems – to get it right,' she wrote. 'I felt terribly frustrated at not having the sensitivity that I had before and I think my boyfriend found it hard. I think I became too over eager to make things alright again.'

Anita felt trapped into having to concentrate on satisfying her partner. 'When I became paralysed I was curious and formed a good sexual relationship with a man. He seemed very satisfied but I was frustrated, particularly after having such a good sexual life with my fiancé before being paralysed. But when you are paralysed you don't have any option when you are a complete lesion, so you go along, or I did, with satisfying your partner.'

The lack of sensation can cause other problems apart from not having an orgasm. Pauline found that: 'because I can't feel all the parts of my body and didn't respond to some touch it used to "kill the moment".' However, Gwen stressed that 'the parts of the body which have been paralysed can still be touched; they're not out of bounds'.

Sometimes partners find our lack of sensation difficult. Naomi's husband: 'says intercourse is not the same knowing that I can't feel anything and prefers not to have intercourse. This has upset me and makes me feel inadequate. He says it isn't important to him any more. I feel it is important and don't think he should stop having intercourse with me and hope gradually to make him realise this. In the meantime we have quite a good sexual relationship without full sexual intercourse.'

Sex and incontinence

Incontinence is one of, if not the most, inhibiting things about paralysis when it comes to having a sexual relationship. Fiona says that she does not even fantasise now about having affairs because of incontinence – 'as we sail into the sunset, who would supply the inco pads?' Some of us have indwelling catheters which either have to be removed before we have sex, or have to be taped out of the way – neither of which is very conducive to spontaneously jumping into bed together. Incontinence pads and plastic pants are also items which we would rather other people did not know about. And even if we do not rely on such aids, and also if we do, we still worry about peeing (or worse) at the most inappropriate moments.

For Abigail, incontinence means that she has no sexual relationship with her husband. And Deborah deliberately decided she did not wish to have a sexual relationship with anyone because of her incontinence. However, she feels very positive about being on her own. 'I live on my own and cope on my own; I have some good friends and don't feel "alone".'

Bridget, paralysed at the age of 32, believes that if this had not happened to her she would have had a sexual relationship with a woman by now, having previously only had heterosexual relationships. Embarrassment about her changed body shape is compounded by the fear of having to explain about incontinence. This, together with the difficulties of entering into a new kind of sexual relationship, has meant that she has felt too inhibited to respond to the women to whom she has been attracted.

Some of us are less bothered about incontinence. Liz advises: 'Don't worry about having to say the words "There's a good chance I might pee on you". If you've got that far he's already accepted you, and will probably give you a wry smile and make a small joke of it . . . and when you do pee on him he won't mind in the slightest and soon you'll be laughing about it and in the end he won't even notice!! You're not the only one with feelings of sexual inadequacy you know!'

Valerie thinks that her initial reluctance to embark on a sexual relationship was due to incontinence but now that she can cope with this independently she feels more confident, and also realises that she possibly felt more sensitive about herself than the person to whom she was attracted.

Contraception

The most common experience related about contraception was the lack of advice – which may, of course, be connected to the notion that we are asexual following paralysis. When advice was offered, there appeared to be major differences of opinion about the Pill and whether it was safe for us to take.

Those of us in our teens when paralysed often missed out on advice about contraception. Marie writes: 'No one in hospital told me about sexual matters or contraception. I suppose because I was only 16. So I had to find out on my own.' Norma was also 16 when she was knocked down by a lorry. 'There was no sexual advice given at all when I was first paralysed, and although we made love before and after my accident happened, I was very innocent about contraception methods.'

However, even when older and in stable relationships or

married at the time of paralysis, we often found that no advice was given regarding contraception. Louise, injured in 1985 and married with two young children, tersely wrote, 'No advice of this nature has ever been given by anyone.' Helen, who was paralysed by a viral infection when she was pregnant with her second child, says, 'No contraceptive advice was ever given by the spinal unit. Luckily I was sub-fertile following paralysis, with no periods and no ovulation, so it wasn't a problem for us.'

It was, however, a problem for Lorna who was paralysed in 1974 when her two sons were aged 5 and 6. 'I think,' she says, 'that the only gap was discussing marital relations and family planning. This resulted in my becoming pregnant within 12 months of my discharge. The pregnancy was terminated.'

Our need for contraceptive advice does not arise just at the time of our paralysis but may become necessary as the years go by and our circumstances change. Geraldine was paralysed when she fell off a swing at the age of 13 in 1978. She has recently married, but: 'I was never given any advice on which type of contraceptive to use because I think my doctor thought that because of my paralysis I shouldn't need any birth control.' Like most of us, Geraldine relied on her own knowledge when taking a decision about contraception, and like many chose the Pill, 'because it was the easiest form of contraceptive on the market.'

In other respects, our experiences of contraceptive devices seem to mirror those of non-disabled women. For example, we have the same tales of silly mistakes on the part of the medical profession when IUDs are inserted. Pamela wrote: 'The doctor who fitted my IUD was so utterly incompetent that within two weeks I was pregnant (a piece of cotton in the uterus, with the coil left outside, is *not* an effective contraceptive).'

When advice *is* given it seems to vary on the subject of the Pill. Some of us were told that we should not take the Pill as paralysis brings about a greater risk of thrombosis; others were told that the Pill is the most suitable form of contraception. Amongst those who sorted things out for themselves, many chose the Pill. For some it has proved ideal; others have experienced side effects that many non-disabled women also experience.

Anita, who was a nurse before she was paralysed, is sceptical about medical advice on contraception. She writes: 'I knew all about the different methods of contraception before I was paralysed. So when I formed a relationship with an able-bodied man we used our own experience. I have never asked a doctor and indeed I don't think I would bother. I know women friends who have been given such ridiculous advice (well you can't even call it advice) from doctors. For my disabled women friends the Pill is said to be taboo because of the risk of thrombosis, yet no research has been done – not at my spinal unit, anyway. The family planning clinics in my county know little about disabled women and very few disabled women go to them.'

Liz was one of those who relied on her own judgement. 'I chose the Pill,' she wrote, 'because it was less elaborate than mechanical methods. After five years I came off it for all the usual reasons. I then took up with natural contraception – using the muco-thermic method, which is much more reliable than the better known "rhythm method". Basically, I made up my own mind about what methods I chose. I've had no problems with either method, but wouldn't advise a "natural" method if you're in the middle of a "grand passion" when the days of "abstinence" wouldn't be appropriate!'

Some of us were told that the 'mini-Pill' would be best for us as there is a diminished risk of thrombosis with this type. Lynne uses the 'mini-Pill', although she is worried about its safety and side effects but thinks that the safest method, from a health point of view, the cap, is too difficult to manage.

Bridget, on the other hand, although she was advised against the cap because a lack of feeling is supposed to make it unsuitable, actually preferred using the cap after being paralysed. 'I didn't like it before my accident as I could feel it and it was uncomfortable. Now I can't feel a thing. I haven't had much occasion to use contraception since my accident, but when I have used it I don't find the lack of feeling any great handicap in using the cap as I can feel with my finger whether it's properly in place.'

'On my own'

Being on our own is a state which some of us are very happy with. Sometimes, as for Lorna, this initially comes about against our wishes. Lorna was married with two small sons when she became paralysed from the shoulders down at the age of 30 in 1974. After some years her husband left her for another woman. She writes: 'When he left, I thought, How do I, a 40-year-old tetraplegic, compete with an attractive 25-year-old physically fit, sexually active woman? The answer was I couldn't! After months of crying, feeling sorry for myself, blaming everything on my wheelchair, I passed off the whole outward charade of myself, and became the real me. I feel happier than I have done in a long time.'

Other women have never thought a sexual relationship to be an important part of their lives. Lindy says: 'Sexuality is something I care little about. A born spinster according to my family!' Ursula's main interest in life, both before and after becoming paraplegic in 1960 at the age of 34, was her job as a research worker. She writes that she didn't really consider whether disability would make any difference to her sexuality, 'but on the other hand I was very interested in my work.' Describing her life, she says, 'Except for the first two years, I've lived on my own and had a full-time job. I've travelled widely. I've had an interesting and, at times, highly entertaining time.'

Sometimes, however, disability and other circumstances have brought about isolation and loneliness. Such is what happened to Violet who was disabled 20 years ago, and for whom widowhood and poverty have brought despair. 'Life is very hard now,' she writes. 'I now live alone in an upstairs flat as I was a rape victim. I never leave it except to go to hospital. I have been widowed 10 years now. I was 44 when my husband died. I suppose I am lonely and frustrated. I have overdosed unsuccessfully. I am very depressed.'

Some of us have found that positive things have come out of disability and feel happy with the way things have worked out. In 1948, Bronwen was working as a nanny when she became paralysed by a virus, transverse myelitis, at the age of 26. She returned to the same job and, when the two children grew older, obtained a job of running a flat for rehabilitating newly disabled women. She gained a great deal of satisfaction from this work and feels that in this way her life has been enhanced by disability. 'I would not have thought of, or been offered, the chance of attempting to help others rehabilitate themselves if I had not been handi-capped myself.' She writes that, following her disability, she did not give any thought to whether her sexuality would be affected. 'People are people to me, not men and women. I find it easier to have close relationships with people of both sexes as I get older.' Indeed, her friends have given her a lot of joy in her life. 'Before I became paralysed, I never knew I had so many friends, in so many different circles, who cared so much. Their support was invaluable. Over the years we have all accepted the ups and downs as they come. I still have most of these friends and have collected a host of others. If that is the result of my disability – and I think that in an indirect way it is – it is a tremendous bonus.'

Bridget feels liberated by her disability from the social pressures to conform to the 'ideal' of a nuclear family. She was a single parent before her accident but 'I believe that if the accident hadn't happened, I would have by now entered into another unsatisfactory sexual relationship. As it is, the opportunities do not present themselves and I am very happy being on my own. I genuinely believe that it is not a case of my making a virtue out of necessity. I love spending time on my own, living in a home which is no one else's but mine. I get an enormous amount of satisfaction and joy from my job, from various types of writing, from reading avidly and from listening to music. And my friends and my daughter provide me with all the closeness in terms of rela-tionships that I want.'

Forming new relationships

Apart from incontinence, there are other barriers to forming new sexual relationships after disability. The attitudes of non-disabled people towards disabled women, which Anita and Pauline describe at the beginning of this chapter – that we should all be asexual – influence the way both men and women relate to us. Lynne 'noticed straight away that men were not treating me as a sexual being (or women either, for that matter).'

Marie is getting very fed up with such attitudes. 'I keep asking myself, what's wrong with me? At first I used to think it was my fault but now I know it is because of the wheel-chair. Men just don't think of me in a sexual way I suppose. But this hurts just as much as if it was because of my person-ality. I suppose men are looking for the "ideal" and I just don't measure up, for whatever reason. I tried answering ads in magazines at one stage and I got on quite well – until I mentioned I was disabled and then heard no more from them. Why is this? Paralysed men don't seem to have the same difficulties – is this because women are more inter-ested in personality than looks?'

Ranjan recognises the part that stereotypes play in her lack of confidence about forming relationships. 'This is largely due to the views held by our society which puts an emphasis on being and looking "perfect" and therefore being able-bodied.'

Forming a new sexual relationship following disability can take a great deal of courage. Annie writes of her initial fears. 'I was afraid of not being able to do anything. Grief-stricken that I might never feel that pleasure again. I was also embarrassed that I might ruin the situation with tears, anger, frustration, incontinence or whatever. At first I did realise my deepest fears, but with the right partner they were turned into beautiful moments of sharing when only the sharing mattered. I could relax and I regained ultimate pleasure in making love. Being single my main fears when forming new relationships were when to explain about the awful pants and pads *and* possible bladder problem, *and* scars *and* (to me) not so wonderful naked body, but it has always worked out alright for me.'

Barbara writes about the combined effects of her own feelings about herself and other people's attitudes to her disability. 'I felt "inferior" to my former self-image. Loss of personal independence hit hard. But I was also affected by how I was perceived by some [members] of the opposite sex. You can still be a friend but the message is "you're a write-off". So I put up a barrier – know me so far but no further because I didn't want to admit to all the horrible aspects of spinal cord injury. Also, needing so much personal help I felt like a child – and children don't have grown-up relationships.'

Charlotte became a paraplegic in 1969 when she was just 17 years old. From her years of experience of disability she writes, 'In making new relationships one needs to be, I think, a little extrovert and make the most of what you have until the person sees you and not the handicap. Then be honest and don't let things like incontinence put you off, but enter it with a feeling of fun – a sense of humour is essential. Sex is fun and there is no reason why a paralysed person should not get as much enjoyment from it as anyone else as long as it is approached in the right spirit. Posture adaptations may have to be made to get and give fulfilment; both women and men must be completely honest and learn which parts of their bodies give them arousal. Intercourse isn't everything and one can be satisfied through the fondling of ears, neck, breasts, etc. Experimentation is essential and is not perverted. Positioning can make a great deal of difference, one position may well give little pleasure to either or both partners but a change can make a great difference. Appliances like catheters can be got round and, if it's a good relationship, they need not be a hindrance to a good loving experience.'

For Kate, disability brought a fundamental change in her sexual identity and a very real liberation from social pressures. 'I have a strong sense of my accident having liberated me when it comes to relationships. I was 19 when I had my accident and I'd grown up with an unthinking expectation of getting married and having numerous children. My immediate reaction in hospital, and for months and years afterwards, was of feeling neutered and completely rejected as a sexual being by men. But I also remember the glimmers of feeling real freedom from society's expectations of me. Society had rejected me but that also meant it didn't have any power over me, either. I didn't have to achieve the role of wife and mother any more.'

Kate continues: 'Even then, I'd got far higher expectations of emotional depth, physical warmth and sensual satisfaction in relationships than the majority of men are capable of. In my early 20s I would have been shocked at the idea that I was gay, but, as I very slowly regained a feeling of being attractive, I also felt free to love whomever I wanted. So that eventually I was able to have my first relationship with a woman without any of the traumas that many of my gay women friends have gone through. I haven't had to face family reaction of "Why haven't you got married?" or society's reaction of "Why haven't you got a man?" – because I'm not *expected* to have one! It's impossible to say what would have happened if I hadn't become paraplegic, but I would most likely have followed the general expectation and got married and now I'd be wondering why I was so dissatisfied with my husband and children. Instead, I am genuinely grateful to my accident for the fact that I have the deepest, most satisfying hopefully lifelong relationship I could ever wish for. And a relationship in which I don't have to conform to ANY roles – I can be ME and loved for that alone.'

As a final word on forming new sexual relationships after injury, Liz stresses the courage of the new partners – 'They have chosen to share the stigma of disability with us. For make no mistake, the world does not accept what they have done lightly but imputes to them motives of sexual inadequacy, kinkiness, or "saintliness" and *not* the transforming power of human love.'

6.

Families and Friends

Families

We each have many roles and relationships in our lives. When we wrote about the effect of our disability on our family, we tended to focus on our role as daughters, and in particular on relationships with our mothers. As with husbands and lovers, the nature of the relationships with parents after our disability is to a large extent determined by previous relationships. Paraplegia and tetraplegia involve what society usually defines as 'severe disability', and this is not something that any parent envisages happening to her or his child. Our injuries bring loss and grief not only to us but also to our families. The reactions of members of our families can provide us with a great deal of support, but can also bring about a lot of pain.

Liz feels disappointed at how her family reacted to her accident. 'All the right things were said and done but I was made to understand from my family that I had "ruined" their lives by courting disaster by climbing mountains. It seemed as if my disability was viewed through the way it had disrupted and affected their lives. I had taken away the daughter they could be proud of and replaced her with a "cripple" that other people would only pity them for being lumbered with. When my father died, the family would often say that my accident had killed him! They liked to martyr themselves to what they thought were my needs and their duty. My biggest mistake was to let my mother control my life – but I couldn't see a way out.'

Eventually, Liz managed to establish a life away from her parents. In contrast, Charlotte, also injured when a teenager, still lives happily with her parents. She describes the impact of her disability on her family and her relationship with her parents and siblings. 'My parents, brother and sister were all devastated. Bills were left unpaid. My father had a minor car accident himself because his mind was on me. My mother gave up marriage counselling. My sister thought I would be bed-ridden. My brother, who was abroad in Africa, shut himself away for a week trying to come to terms [with the situation] and work it out. He was reluctant to talk to anyone and was depressed. All this I found out much later. When I came home, at first it was a great strain on everyone to behave normally, and when my brother got home 18 months later he was at first shocked with the reality and didn't know how to react.'

Charlotte continues: 'Now, 15 years later, I am treated as an integral part of the family as if nothing had happened, apart from cursing the chair (not me) when it gets in everyone's way. We have all learnt to adapt and have been thinking of ways round problems that the chair and my inability to stand or walk create, e.g. sailing – ways of getting in and out of the boat with the least amount of hassle and how to reach the upper floor of the club house which has two staircases which are at an acute angle wth treads so narrow the chair won't rest on them. Within the home I'm part of the family and expected to do my whack.'

We have different feelings about whether or not our families have accepted our disability. Annie writes that: 'Initially my parents expressed total shock, grief, disbelief, etc. They didn't know how to cope with the situation and we had many frustrated arguments. Now (six years later), to my private hurt and anger they've accepted it and cannot understand why I still feel desperate times of grief and suffering.'

On the other hand, Celia says, 'My mother is still deeply saddened by my accident over 20 years ago. I feel that I have to protect her from my disability as she cannot really come to terms with it. I ask myself why I should expect her to – how I would react if it happened to my son.'

Indeed, many of our families find it very difficult to relate to us immediately after our injury, and some find that their feelings about our disability continue to get in the way of their relationship with us. This can be very painful. Sandra writes of how her disability has affected her relationships with members of her family. 'They were uncomfortable in my presence at first and plainly did not know what to say to me. . . . My mother was frightened to come and visit because she has an irrational fear of all things to do with disabilities of any sort . . . As the years have gone by they treat me just the same as anyone else. My sisters are at ease with me now, although when I see them they are rather inclined to say "Don't you look well?!" as if they do not expect me to. My mother, too, has adjusted to my disability, though she tends to treat me as a little girl at times. It took her a couple of years to accept me as I am.'

Disability can make the process of becoming independent from our parents more difficult. Pamela, who was in her early 20s when she had a car accident, continues to be exasperated by her mother's attitude to her disability and her own feelings about accepting help from her mother cause conflict between them. Immediately after her accident, her parents very much wanted to look after her but Pamela felt that her mother was being: 'over-protective and this caused conflict between my mother and my husband which still endures. My mother expected that my husband would not be able to cope with my disability because he was young (22). She almost wanted him not to, so that she could take me home and look after me herself. This would have been disastrous, because I would never have regained my independence. My mother now lives with us (following my father's death in 1979) and she still treats me like an invalid – if she sees me limping down to the clothes-line with the laundry basket, she tries to grab it, saying, "Why didn't you ask me to help you?" I find this very hard to endure and I probably accept less help from her than most able-bodied women do from their mothers, because I am still trying to show her that I CAN MANAGE.'

If we rely on our family for personal care this can interfere with relationships, particularly if those relationships are strained anyway, as Liz describes. 'When I first came home from hospital, I had to rely on my family to "wait" on me in terms of meals, cups of tea, making beds and doing my washing and reaching things from inaccessible places – I found this frustrating because I could see the only reason I couldn't do these things was because the house and the way it was laid out wasn't suitable. Other people doing necessary things never bothered me but impatience while I would laboriously do something upset me, like mother wanting to put my shoes on because I took too long – that sort of thing. There is never any resentment or humiliation involved when help is given by a professional – somehow this is not the case when it's family. I never felt any reluctance to have a hand to an inaccessible loo from a professional; I intensely disliked the same help from my family. They brought something murky to it – as if you were a child again.'

Lynne, on the other hand, has had a very different experience. When she first came out of hospital, her mother provided all the personal care she needed as a tetraplegic, and they maintained their close relationship through this period. 'She gave up her job, and although I wasn't happy that she had had to do this, I made sure that she knew it was only a temporary set up. She took up work again when I started at university and in the holidays, [my holidays] luckily, she didn't work, as she was working at a primary school. My three sisters and friends were also very supportive and helped me with personal care. Accepting the fact that I was dependent on others for such mundane tasks was very hard, and still is sometimes, especially when carers expect eternal thanks for their "charity". I never had this problem with family or friends, but [I did] with a few of the carers I have come across at college and since then. My mother has always been a great support and encouraged me to take the next step in life (and sometimes pushed me when I needed it – no pun intended). My accident brought us closer. My father found it more difficult to accept as he was living away from Mum and had remarried. He still feels guilty and is over-protective.'

Isabel recognises that often we grow away from our families for reasons which have nothing to do with disability. She found life after her injury very difficult to begin with as her parents treated her like a baby. 'It was hard on my family as they had virtually no help or counselling to come to terms with it. They now recognise me as someone who is active and does things, and now I think it is personality differences that keep us apart rather than my disability.'

Disability can mean that our families feel that we cannot fulfil the same role as we could when we were able-bodied. Carol writes: 'Although an issue was never made of it, I feel my parents were very disappointed with what happened, especially as it considerably limited my marriage prospects and hence production of grandchildren. My family was over-protective at the beginning and I had to leave home soon after leaving hospital so that I could develop to my full potential. My parents are still disappointed, but I'm living abroad now and doing well so they are pleased with my successes. They would still have liked grandchildren, though, and preferred that I was complete.'

Molly, married with two young children, found that her mother-in-law was worried that her 'son and grandchildren were going to suffer irreparable neglect. She now has more confidence in my abilities to keep the family fed and alive, but still feels sorry for her son who could have had a "nice normal girl".'

On the other hand, Moira (disabled in 1953 when she was 20 years old) found that her role within the family remained much the same. 'My family were always very supportive and didn't treat me any differently than before. We now have my mother and father living here with us. They are getting old so in a sense we look after them, now.'

Sometimes injury was part of an event which tore a family apart, as it was for Ranjan whose family even so gave her tremendous support. 'My family, that is my extended family, especially my grandmother and my father, suffered a great deal as my mother had died in the same accident. They all had to look after me and they did that with lots of love and care, but it caused them a lot of anguish and pain.'

Nicola was also a child when she was paralysed and, unlike Ranjan who left most of her family behind when she came to England to a spinal unit, has maintained a close relationship with her parents. 'I think my paralysis has brought my family closer together. We pull together as a team and always try to work together. At the same time, we all lead our own separate lives. My family have, along with myself, grown up with my disability.'

The trauma of accident or illness can make someone much more special to those that love them, as Leila found. 'My family have stuck by me through everything. They haven't changed, being wonderful people and are happy because I'm happy. I am a bit special though, I think, to both my parents, having survived a broken back.'

Friends

The dramatic change in our lives sometimes brings friends closer together. Bridget found this with her circle of women friends who formed a 'support group' for her after her accident. 'We have become closer over the years. Part of our experience has been the realisation that we are all getting older (we are in our 30s and 40s) and that personal tragedies (major or minor) are becoming increasingly common. We all need each other and our friendship is very important to me.'

On the other hand, Barbara became aware that some of her friends, while quite happy to see her in her own home, were not comfortable about being out in public with her. The public image of disability, which we have to cope with every time we go outside the front door, can be hard for friends to confront.

We have all found that some friends that we had at the time of our injury have stayed friends and some have disappeared out of our lives. Sometimes this is because our values, interests and priorities have changed, as Anita describes. 'My life has taken on a different direction and, although I'm not pleased about being paralysed, I'm glad that my life changed direction. I feel a more valued person now than I did before and I like myself as a person better, too. It is hard to explain that to your friends or family. Always with friends, the ones who didn't have those values when you were able-bodied, drift away and the ones who did stay with you all along the way. I always wish I were more mobile to help them when they have a crisis – that's when I feel angry about the chair and paralysis, that freedom just to go quickly to a friend is gone. My former work colleagues have developed relationships all over the place so I see them if they are passing, but the ones that were close keep in touch. I have more close friends now than I ever had in my life before and I feel very warm about that; it's a really good feeling.'

We all strive to re-establish as much of our previous lives as possible after injury, and friendships are an important part of this continuity. The initial reaction of friends, most of whom are totally unfamiliar with disability, is an important hurdle to overcome, and those friendships which survive are of great value to us. Sometimes, however, it seems that friends reach a stage where they no longer think about the consequences of being disabled, which may mean that they fail to understand how our needs and concerns are, to at least some extent, different from theirs. Rosalind, for example, feels that some of her friends do not appreciate the physical difficulties of daily living for a paraplegic. 'Some people have got so used to me being independent that they don't realise what a strain it is sometimes. If I tell them, they sometimes brush it aside with "You're doing so well", etc. When I'm going through a bad patch and need more help, I find it hard not to feel that I am making a fuss.'

Finding friends

There can often be barriers to forming new friendships, mainly stemming from people's ignorance and fear of disability but also from our own feelings and lack of confidence. Geraldine writes: 'In the early days I was very aware of my chair and I think this affected my confidence. Also, people did not know how to approach or talk to me. I no longer think about the chair. If I am meeting people for the first time I think that they will either accept me as I am or they won't. If they don't, I don't have to meet them again.'

Helen, like many of us, has now learnt to overcome other people's shyness and lack of knowledge. 'At first I was very reluctant to go anywhere new – I would rather spend time with people who I'd known previously. I was embarrassed at having to remain seated all the time. I am much more confident now having realised that a disabled person usually has to make the first move to make new friends or start a conversation.'

Liz writes of how, over the years, she has learnt to deal with other people's attitudes. 'That people viewed me as a "cripple" greatly shocked and hurt me. You so often get treated as a lesser being that it is commendable to be kind to that this disturbs your psyche into becoming cynical and very wary. I found people wanted either to pity me or put me on a pedestal. It took time to learn to see this coming and diffuse it. On the whole very few people seem to treat you normally and when they do you blossom under it and friendship follows. Now I don't ever expect easy friendship in everyday intercourse. I'm careful never to give anyone the chance to accuse me of a chip on the shoulder that I don't have. I smile, am polite and friendly but keep a dispassionate eye on all social gatherings. Anyone who is without prejudice or preconceptions will see me for what I am and make friends if they want to. I see no point in trying to "convert" the patronising and the prejudiced. I don't need their sort of friendship.'

Norma was only 16 when she was injured and found that she lacked confidence in the early years of disability. 'I hid myself in the comfort of my family. Things have changed to a certain extent. I am alright meeting strangers when I am with someone I know but I get very self-conscious when left to my own devices. However, people's attitudes are much better now. You are not made to feel a freak and once you get talking to people they soon accept you for the person that you are.'

Unfortunately, ignorance means that people sometimes

think we are disabled in ways in which we are not disabled. Elsie regrets how 'I felt like a second-class citizen mainly because people seemed too frightened to talk to me and treated me as a mental case'. Things are better now as 'I tend to make people talk and try to get them to understand I am a "normal" person'. Many of us recognise that we have to take the lead in interacting with other people. This can be difficult, as Rosalind says, 'I find it hard work trying to put people at their ease and trying to be more confident than I really am.'

Ignorance can also mean that each new person whom we get to know has to be 'educated' about disability. This can be tedious, as Linda points out. 'The problem is that one has to go through the same process each time one meets new acquaintances.' Sometimes, other people's activities exclude anyone with a mobility disability. Nicola wrote, 'I have made few new friends over the past years. I find this a difficult task, not because I do not try, but I find that young people of my own age naturally want to experience life to its fullest, which often discounts someone in a wheelchair.'

Other people's reactions to us can prompt us to behave in ways which make forming new friendships more difficult. Vicky says that, in the early days of her disability, she was too defensive to allow people past 'the ironmongery of the wheelchair'. Now she feels that 'I am so independent and do so much in my life that I think I frighten some people away'.

Isabel, who writes elsewhere in this book of how positive she now feels about herself after 30 years of disability, describes how her feelings about making new friends have changed over the years. 'I have many more friends now, with or without disability, women and men, gay and heterosexual, and I find it easier to make new friends, perhaps because I'm involved in so many groups. I do meet people who are nervous about disability and with some of them it's impossible to overcome their fears and so any friendship stops dead. I find I don't feel rejected in these cases. Instead, I feel sorry for them because it's clear they will have a very bad time if or when they have a disability themselves.'

7.

Education and Occupation

A disability such as spinal cord injury can happen to anyone at any stage of their lives. This is reflected in both the wide age range amongst the women who returned our questionnaire and in the variety of occupations in which we were engaged at the time of paralysis. This chapter looks at our educational and occupational experiences, at unpaid and paid work, both inside and outside the home, and at how disability affected these occupations.

To be disabled means a high risk of unemployment and also difficulties in getting the education and/or training we want. This is partly because we are directly discriminated against – there being no law against such discrimination. Another reason is the indirect discrimination which occurs because jobs, and education or training, which are potentially open to us are in fact not available because of the lack of facilities, whether physical access, toilets or enabling equipment. A few occupations, of course, would be completely impossible for us to do under any circumstances, but many which seem impossible are only like this because of the lack of necessary resources.

Another limiting factor is whether or not we have the same energy and/or incentive as we did before we were paralysed to prove ourselves in the world of paid work. Some of us are proud that we have continued in paid work following our disability, but some of us value achievements and life styles which cannot be measured by the conventional criteria of status and income.

Returning to school

Seventeen of us were at school at the time of injury, and only five were able to return to the same school. Eileen described herself as a 'horrible rebellious teenager, convinced that school was a complete waste of time'. She continued: 'My main ambition was to leave school at the earliest opportunity, earn a lot of money fast and then go off and wander around the world.' She became tetraplegic as a result of a road traffic accident in 1961. 'No one knew what to do with a tetraplegic 14-year-old so no one suggested that I return to school or try to find work. At that time this situation suited me perfectly. Later I regretted my lack of education but by then I was too busy with other things to do anything about it.' She did not return to school and has never worked outside the home. She writes: 'In the main, I am satisfied with my achievements. I manage 90 per cent of the housework which I feel compensates my parents to some extent for the help they give me. I serve on several local committees involved with disability, campaign locally for better access and facilities and, as I have never had any burning ambition to work for my living, this makes me feel I'm achieving something with my life.'

Thirteen-year-old Dora also did not return to school. In 1937 she 'was in a general hospital for three months then moved to a children's hospital and remained there for two years. I had physio and they got me walking on crutches.' She carried on with her education in hospital. However she then 'left the children's hospital, went home for a few months, then the war came, so I was evacuated with other disabled children. When I was past my sixteenth birthday I had to leave. As my father had got rid of our home, as he didn't have a wife, I had to go to a hospital for incurables in which I remained for 16 years.' She reflects on this period of her life. 'As I was so capable of looking after myself, and also others less able to, I thought, what a waste of a life.' Since then, however, Dora has been married and then worked in domestic work. Later she trained and then worked as a punch card operator for 16 years before retiring.

For those who continued their education, the usual option offered has been to change schools. This has been primarily because of problems of physical access to school buildings but also because sometimes 'ordinary' education is no longer considered suitable for us. Amy, paralysed when she was 12 in 1977, said, 'I couldn't go back to my old school which I would love to have done. I had to go to a special school.' This meant leaving family and friends, as Melanie also had to do. She was 14 when she became a tetraplegic in 1979 and wrote, 'I was sent to a rehabilitation unit and then to a special boarding school after five months. I think this was far too soon [for me] to leave my parents.'

Harriet lives in Kenya and was paralysed in 1978 when she was 17. 'I was lucky to get a school not very far from home where I joined at the beginning of 1980 as a boarder. This was all possible due to sheer luck and determination. Minor problems such as small stairs to classes were sorted out through co-operation of the headmistress with the social workers.' She did her O and A levels at this school and then went on to college to train as an aviation communicator.

Charlotte had no difficulty returning to the same school after she was paralysed in a car accident in 1969 when she was 17. Luckily, the school was a single storey building and the few steps were ramped and a toilet converted. But Caroline, injured in 1982 at the age of 16, had a struggle to return to her A level studies. 'The education authority were keen to send me to a special residential school . . . However, through the work of my school, school doctor and commuity occupational therapist, I was able to return to school in September 1983. The only expense incurred was the provision of a Gimson Stairmate, the building of a few ramps and the knocking of two toilets into one. The education authority also financed a locally run group who have been coming to empty my leg bag and give me a lift during the lunch hour.'

Being a student

Ten of us were at university or college when we became

disabled. Three were unable to return, two because of lack of access. Isabel wrote: 'The college was totally inaccessible so I gave up that career. In fact, everyone else's expectation of me was now lower than before and nothing else was suggested.'

Elaine's college was also inaccessible. 'My life was totally changed. I could have gone back to college 10 years later but I had lost the urge by that time. I've achieved nothing.' For Avril, however, it was the level of paralysis which prevented her returning to her studies. She broke her neck while trampolining in 1980, and the loss of the use of her arms and hands meant that she could not continue her course in textiles and PE. Although she now runs a small gift shop, she writes: 'I do not feel stretched mentally and so I am not totally satisfied.'

Six of us who were at university or college when we became paralysed were able to continue in higher education studies, although two had to change colleges. Elise, who was a 20-year-old art student when she became a paraplegic, wrote: 'I stayed in the same job, painting. Still having the use of my hands, it made no difference. The only problem is carrying the pictures.' She continues: 'I am proud I achieved my degree but have had no real job since, just sold pictures privately and had the odd exhibition.'

Vicky, who became tetraplegic in 1974 when she was 19, switched to computer studies when she returned to college. 'I was studying music but could no longer do the practical work or get into the department, so I had to switch to another subject. I had to completely rethink the direction I was heading in as my original hopes/plans were no longer feasible. At least I was injured at a stage where it was relatively easy to change direction. I would not have dreamt of a career in computing before but have done very well in a field where sitting down is no handicap at all. I am now completely satisfied career-wise, although I would have chosen an occupation that involved a little more movement and meeting people.'

Christine had been studying modern languages when a fall at the seaside left her walking with sticks and knee calipers.

She was uncertain at first about continuing with her intention of becoming a teacher. 'I returned to college, but when I finished my degree I did wonder whether I could cope with being a teacher. So I did a degree in experimental psychology in order to be a psychologist, probably an educational psychologist. But then to do that I needed to do teacher training anyway, and once I started teaching I never wanted to move on to being an educational psychologist. I did cope with teaching OK and I'm now a college of education lecturer.'

Tessa completed her degree after she became paraplegic. She then got a job in a research institute as a mathematician. She wrote: 'The only way in which my paralysis perhaps affected my choice was that I tried institutes near home first. I do not know if I would have done otherwise. I wrote to them on the "I'm me, what can I do for you? Are you interested?" principle.'

A number of those injured while at school went on to higher education, including Nasreen who is proud of her achievement in becoming 'the first person in a wheelchair in Jordan to complete university'. Thirteen of the 25 women who have completed schooling or further or higher education since injury are now in full-time work. Two are in part-time work and nine are not in paid work. Five of those in full-time work are high level tetraplegics.

Getting a job

As newly disabled women we generally had very little help and guidance in finding a job. Most of us never met Disablement Resettlement Officers, and those that did had little complimentary to say about them. They were described as 'useless' and 'a nightmare'. Angela, for example, had worked for a publisher in an old, inaccessible building. She visited the DRO 'who restricted looking for vacancies to my local area and complained that I was over-qualified'.

Another 'over-qualified' woman, Cynthia, was a teacher and wrote: 'I got no help from the DRO. I was given a

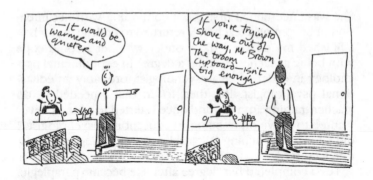

factory job by him.' Cora, too, wrote of her experience.
'When I was looking for work – I am professionally trained
– the DRO said he could get me a job in the packaging
department of a factory if I could walk just a few steps. I had
explained I was a complete paraplegic.'

Liz could not return to her previous job when she became
a paraplegic at the age of 18. She wrote: 'I was sent to work
within a few weeks of discharge from the spinal unit by an
appalling DRO who insisted I would vegetate if I remained at
home. I felt ill and was desperate for rest and calm – not
things you get in a spinal unit. The lack of an accessible loo
was lightly dismissed by the DRO and everyone else. My
mother to her credit protested at the whole idea, but we
were both shouted down. The offer of a job – "not everyone is willing to take on someone like you" – was too good
to miss. I was made to feel guilty and ungrateful if I didn't
take it. In consequence of which my full recovery was, I'm
sure, delayed for several years and all for a paltry wage and
the dubious therapy of being in work.'

Some of us who have sought jobs following our disability
have found it difficult to overcome discriminatory attitudes
towards our abilities. Monica had worked in a solicitor's
office before she had children. Her husband was killed in
the car crash which left her paralysed in 1967, when her
children were very young. She wrote: 'When the children
were old enough for me to return to work I found it almost
impossible to get anything.' She picked up any work going –

'I worked one day a week for POSSUM (an organisation providing electronic equipment for disabled people). Then a
friend who is a retired solicitor gave me his personal work to
do. I also worked one day a week for an accountant. Then
by chance a friend saw an advert in the paper for a clerk
neded for a nursery for disabled children. I now have that
job working four days a week.'

Celia, who walks with crutches, experienced both direct
and indirect discrimination when she tried to return to
office work when her son was old enough. 'I tried for jobs,
but it's Catch 22. Mention disability and they don't want to
know; don't mention it until you get an interview and they
still aren't interested.' She eventually got a job but then had
to give it up because 'access and parking were insurmountable problems. It was a very hilly locality and there were
masses of stairs in the old building with no lift.'

Unfortunately, the experience of Marie is not very common. She is a T5 paraplegic and took up office work with the
Civil Service after her injury. She commented: 'The Civil
Service have been good to me and have not shown any discrimination against me. They also try and accommodate
your special needs. But not all employers would do this.'

Taking up work again

Some of us who had been in paid employment before injury
felt that returning to work was something which motivated
us towards recovery. Olivia had been working as a secretary
and looked forward to going back. 'The personnel officer
[from work] visited me in the spinal unit in the first few
weeks of my being admitted to tell me that without question
there would be a job for me to go back to. This was a great
incentive and I promised to be back within six months. And
I achieved my goal! I was discharged from the spinal unit on
the Friday and went back to work on the Monday.'

Not all of us had such sympathetic employers. Bridget's
employer, a local education authority, sacked her when
they found out that she was in a wheelchair as a result of her

accident in 1983. 'The accident happened at the end of the summer term and they waited until the first week of the autumn term to tell me that my contract was void. My union got me my job back, although even they didn't take the case up until they realised that such action had implications for other teachers. A friend from work staged a solitary picket of the education committee, handing out a leaflet headed "What Price Progress with Humanity?" (Progress with Humanity being the motto of this "equal opportunities" employer.)'

Rosemary has also had problems with her employer, a major bank. She had been working as a secretary in a branch 15 miles away from her home, but following her paralysis accepted downgrading to a shorthand typist in a branch where her husband worked. 'I had trouble getting the boss to accept that I was capable of a full day's work and I felt he was forever watching over me waiting for me to make a mistake.'

Rachel, who works for an estate agent, complained: 'I was put into a rear office so as not to disturb clients. My boss was afraid they would prefer to talk about me instead of business.'

Some of us have also encountered difficulties with work colleagues. Fiona, a doctor, was the senior partner in a three-woman general practice at the time of her paralysis as a result of a spinal tumour in 1981. 'My partners wanted me to retire. I had suggested going back for six months and seeing how it went – I had paid for locums while I was off. I also suggested job-sharing. There was a long and unhappy legal wrangle. I was excluded from all business decisions, etc. In the end I was invited to join another practice. I moved, and that is going very well. I have more patients than before and I'm teaching students and GP trainees again.'

Sometimes these misconceived attitudes drove us forward. This was true of Ursula, a research worker, who wrote, 'The director didn't like women, much less one who was paralysed and could cope. How I hated that man! But it did drive me to do many things that otherwise I might not have done.'

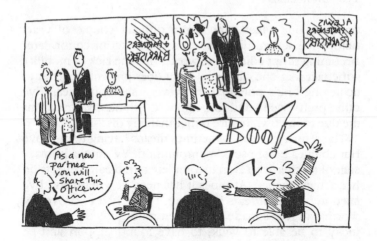

On the other hand, several of us had, and have, anxieties and doubts about our promotion prospects. Judith had qualified for hotel and catering management before her car accident. She says: 'I was unable to take a job in that field and I have been employed as a clerical officer with responsibility for therapeutic diets at the local hospital since returning to work after the accident. Now I have cold feet about pursuing a hope to go into management. Because catering is a very practical job I had to change my thinking completely.'

Many jobs involving manual work can still be done following disability. For example, Janet worked as a raincoat machinist before her accident in 1961. A widow with two sons, she could have returned to work since, although she can no longer use a treadle, she can use a machine with button control. She writes, however, 'I could not have been employed because toilet facilities were not suitable.'

Nursing is one job which involves a lot of manual work which would prove impossible for a paraplegic or tetraplegic to return to (unless it was to nursing education). Jane was an SRN and writes: 'Being paralysed means I can never return to my profession.' There are other circumstances, too, where lack of mobility can be a major handicap because of the nature of the job. Alison, for example, had been a director's assistant in television drama but this job 'had to be done on one's feet'. She had a difficult couple of years before she settled down as an assistant script editor, later becoming script editor. She wrote: 'It's the lack of mobility – the fact that one can't run – that does present a barrier to achieving one's potential. However,' she continues, 'I've done pretty well – and to be honest, I think my limitations are due to my own nature rather than my disability.'

The return to work sometimes means having to re-prove our abilities before seeking promotion. Yvonne, a primary school teacher who is an incomplete tetraplegic, reflects on her achievements. 'At times it has been very hard and I've shed my share of tears in private. I have had to prove my worth and it has made promotion more difficult. I was so lucky to be able to walk, to have found support and be determined to the point of obstinacy.'

Gillian taught PE, biology and outdoor pursuits in a secondary school before her climbing accident which left her a paraplegic. When the time came to return to work, 'I was offered chances to teach in schools for physically handicapped or educationally subnormal children, or retraining in a different subject with no firm job offer at the end. I pushed to be allowed to go to a junior school and the union helped enormously in this field – I doubt I would have succeeded without them. I now teach in a junior school as an assistant to the teacher. My career has been affected quite a lot by my accident. I'm not yet satisfied with my achievements. I've been taken on by a school to gain experience and only now am I anywhere near getting my own class of children.'

Hilary, a health visitor, was also unable to return to her previous occupation and was prepared to accept employment at a lower status in the hope of being able to work her way back. 'This meant forgetting the qualifications I had and settling for a lesser paid job of clinic clerk. The fact that someone was prepared to employ me was reward in itself. My career has certainly been affected by my paralysis. I have progressed through part-time clinic clerk to teaching health education and human biology in school to my present job of full-time day centre organiser.'

The statistics illustrate our employment difficulties, some of which stem from direct or indirect discrimination. Of the 103 of us who were in full-time paid employment prior to disability, 48 did not return to work and 39 took up different paid employment (three of these working from home). Fifteen of us who had been working full-time before our disability changed to part-time work after injury.

Opening doors

Some of us, unable to return to our previous jobs, chose to change direction. This often meant retraining, and for some there have been positive benefits in rethinking our working lives. Carol had been a biological researcher in Bolivia. At first she stayed in the same field of work, albeit in London, but then did a course in librarianship and information science. After a while, she changed direction again and trained as a social worker, working for several years with a local authority and then with a voluntary agency. In 1976 Carol won a Churchill Travelling Fellowship which, she says, 'opened many doors. I have enjoyed the challenges in the zigzag course I've pursued and am still changing, latterly doing a management course.'

Someone else whose life has dramatically changed as a result of paralysis is Paula, who had been working as a hospital clerk before her husband stabbed her in the back. Fearing his release from prison, she emigrated with her six-year-old twins to Australia. She writes: 'I have now almost completed a degree in teaching and will shortly be a fully trained primary school teacher. I would never have thought that I would be where I am now had I not been attacked, divorced and come to Australia.'

Linda was forced to change course when, following her car accident, the college of education where she worked refused to let her go into schools to supervise her students 'because I might disrupt classes'. When the college then amalgamated with another and moved to an unsuitable site, she retrained to be a solicitor. 'It has proved to be a good choice although I miss teaching languages dreadfully.' She has progressed in directions other than work, although there are obstacles here as well. 'It has curbed my ambition. I am fairly content with my position and prefer to achieve progress for disabled people and contribute to the community, generally outside work. I had intended to try to become an MP but find the political process very tiring. I feel I could contribute effectively at Westminster but constituency electioneering poses enormous problems for a wheelchair user.'

When a career depends on our physical ability, paralysis can be particularly heartbreaking. Gina has taken a while to develop an alternative direction after breaking her neck in 1973. She had been a dancer until an accident on stage when she was 22 years old. She relates her experience: 'Obviously I couldn't dance any more, but I wasn't interested in teaching or choreographing from my wheelchair. I couldn't think of anything that I wanted to do other than dance, which was a big problem. It was very frustrating, still being connected with dancers as friends and watching performances, etc. I have only recently been back to college to do costume design and am now a freelance designer. This enables me to work from home mainly, but I also go to watch rehearsals and get involved with the production side. I need to be creative again. I wish it had happened sooner, i.e. finding a different career. I am not as ambitious to have a successful career in design as I was in dance.'

Another tetraplegic, Barbara, could not return to teaching as her level of disability prevented her taking the post which was offered to her. She was then offered a post in the school library. This has had advantages as well as disadvantages. 'It's a unique situation,' she wrote. 'I can use my teaching skills . . . There is tremendous variety and I have had a free hand in how the job has developed. It is very enjoyable. But it is not a career.'

Sarah's experience, although very different, still serves to illustrate the changes some of us have undergone in our lives. A member of a religious order at the time of her accident, she writes, 'As a result of becoming paralysed, life was changed completely. Before my accident it seemed as if I was set to spend the rest of my life as a religious sister but I was not solemnly professed so was not accepted back into the order. Instead I am now very happily married with a home of our own.'

Coping

Some of us have found the combined pressures of work and disability too much of a strain. Cynthia, for example, has had to take early retirement. 'My job as a home economics teacher became physically too difficult for me. I would have been able to continue teaching in a non-practical subject and in looking back think I should have done a course in another subject after my accident. However, I am happy that I did persevere and got a great deal of satisfaction out of being able to hold down a demanding job.'

Marie, who had been doing clerical work before her motor bike accident, also writes of the difficulties of holding down a full-time job. She now works for the Civil Service in the same type of work and perseveres in spite of the difficulties. 'I do find working full-time very tiring and I always seem to be rushing against time. It takes me longer to do things and so I cannot cope with too much pressure at work. However, my colleagues do understand this. But I still do my full job and pull my weight. I make no concessions to my disability.'

Charlotte, injured when she was still at school, went to work as a full-time receptionist when her education finished. 'The toilet was unsuitable but I coped for three to four years before my health broke down. This took the form of tonsil trouble and I had to have them out. Now whether my paralysis was the major factor, manifesting itself through other parts of the body, I'm not sure, but I have never since then managed more than 10 hours work a week before becoming ill in some way or another.' In spite of these limitations on her working life, Charlotte is pleased with the work she does. 'I now work for DIAL Essex [a disability organisation], normally six hours a week, and find this highly satisfying and fulfilling. I also do lecturing to all ages, the last major feat being to speak on disablement to 200 fourth formers in batches of 30 at one of our local comprehensives. I also give talks to nurses and doctors – in fact, a wide spectrum of people. I believe that having had to find out about everything the hard way, being outgoing and all that I've done since my accident does at least leave me fairly content with my lot.'

Some of us have major physical problems which prevent us going out to work. Mavis, who became paralysed over a number of years, gradually found that she could only sit for up to three-and-a-half to four hours in her chair. She had gained an accountancy qualification in the hope of doing freelance work but found this was difficult to get as she couldn't leave her home. She now spends most of her time in her bed, but writes, 'I have enough work to fill my two-hour day permitted. I enjoy and find it very rewarding, especially since I have been bedfast. I live in the lounge and therefore I'm in touch with everything which takes place or is organised within my house.'

Pain, which so often is an important part of living with spinal cord injury, can restrict our working lives, particularly when combined with the tiredness caused by the sheer physical effort of life in a wheelchair. Rosalind certainly feels that her working life has been inhibited by disability. She writes: 'I think that my career has been affected by my paralysis in that I don't have enough stamina to do the job properly. When I returned to work I was working five days a week, with short hours. About two years ago I changed to a four-day week as I needed more time for personal care, shopping, chores and relaxation. I have bad root pain and it becomes unbearable when I get overtired. Working shorter hours has affected my chances of promotion. I was pleased that I did go back to work, but now feel that I hold the job down with a struggle.'

Tessa, having started off so well in her job as a mathematician, now writes, 'Recently the strain of coping with an extremely demanding job and life in general got too much and I had to give up work.' She was 20 when she became a paraplegic in 1979, and echoes a sentiment which it took

Liz, injured in 1969, some years to express: 'some paraplegics, especially if we had other injuries, find the whole 9–5
routine plus travelling too much to cope with. I really don't
think every paraplegic is up to it.' Liz went on to identify the
dilemma in which we are placed by society's expectations.
'Society makes it next to impossible for us to get employment that pays enough to live on, unless we've been trained
in a profession. Therefore the emphasis of self-esteem and
respect placed upon being in work (as if housework isn't
work) is damaging to those who can't work outside the
home. We have to tolerate all manner of snide and patronising remarks from the self-righteous employed. We are
judged by what we do and not what we are. It is yet another
bitter pill to swallow.' She stresses the value of work in the
home. 'I've always been able to pull my weight in the household I've run and been successful in the despised role of
chief cook and bottle washer. I don't find it demeaning. It is
a craft in its own right and frees other people to have careers
and be employed.'

Out of the rat race

There can be no denying the effect that spinal cord injury
has had upon all our lives. For some it has been devastating
and for others it has provided an opportunity to reassess
values and look at achievements. Cora was: 'at a crossroads
as to which way my life and profession was going to go
when my accident occurred. It has never bugged me that I
never achieved the professional heights. In fact (to myself) I
have been able to use my paraplegia as an excuse for not
hitting the "top". I'm now considered by myself and others
as a whole person rather than a person plus a profession.'

Isabel feels there are positive things which resulted from
being disabled. 'I think what I do now is completely the
result of my disability. I do the administration for a national
lesbian women's group and I work with several other disability related groups, e.g. a drop-in group, an employment
group, a sexuality group as well as non-disability related
ones, e.g. a writers' group, vegetarian group and lesbian and

gay campaigning groups. I'm happy with what I'm doing – I can't ever feel complete satisfaction because there is always so much more to be done and not enough time to do it. I'm pleased I've become a more positive person and it's good to meet so many different people in their different areas of voluntary work. It can be maddening but never boring.'

Some of us have thought carefully about whether we really wanted to struggle to carry on a working life, as if our disability had not happened – and concluded that we did not want to do so. Libby was injured in 1980. She is an incomplete tetraplegic, walking with a stick and with little use in her left hand. She walks very slowly and tires easily. 'I don't want a full-time job,' she writes, 'or a very pressurised job, now. I have just left university and am looking for a job but it is a rather half-hearted search. I feel that having to take everything at a slower pace, now, I look at things differently. I don't feel inclined to join in the commercial rat race. I have no ambition as far as climbing the career ladder goes. I feel satisfied in that I managed to get to university after a long gap, and in spite of difficulties such as a much reduced writing speed, but frustrated in that jobs such as teaching in Third World countries, which I would now be interested in, are out of the question. I know some disabled people do amazing things and with worse disabilities than mine, but I don't have the confidence or determination to do the same.'

Sarah, whose life changed so radically when she left her religious order following her disability, reflects: 'Is one ever really satisfied with what one has achieved? In many respects I would apply the old adage – "could do better". But I am content with my life as a married woman, sharing in a deep, fruitful and rewarding relationship, looking after our home, while contributing a little towards the more general fellowship in the wider world.' She continued: 'For me it has been fight all the way; some hard struggles, many funny incidents, warmth and support from my fellow creatures, remembering particularly the importance of giving and taking, as well as a fair share of heartbreak. Sometimes, one can "stand" in the trench lines and muse at those creatures who call themselves normal.'

8.

Being a Mother

Eighty-six of us had children at the time of our injury and 27 had children under the age of five. Three women were pregnant at the time of injury. Twenty of us had children following paralysis.

'My two-year-old didn't recognise me'

A major concern for those of us who had young children at the time of injury was how our children reacted to separation from us. The most usual period of time spent in hospital was five to six months, but in fact the length varied from three months to two years. For many this was a time of feeling cut off from our children, heartbreak at the break in the relationship and sometimes intense jealousy of the substitute carer. Young children and babies are very pragmatic creatures who respond to whoever looks after them. Our children therefore bonded with their substitute carers and many of us felt usurped and betrayed, a trauma which at times was felt to be a greater tragedy than the injury itself, particularly if we were not happy with the care that was provided. For example, Lorna wrote: 'I think my concern for the boys [aged 5 and 6] was more traumatic than any of my own medical problems.'

However, all of us found that once we were home our relationships with our child or children were re-established; we became 'Mum' again and within months it was as if we had never been away. For most of the younger children, as they got older there was no memory of separation or of their mother being any different.

Young children were most commonly looked after by partners (in 13 cases), mothers or sisters (in 24 cases) or a combination of the two (21 cases). In only two cases did statutory agencies take over total care of the children; in six other instances statutory agencies were involved together with partners and/or relatives.

Helen had a daughter aged 13 months when she had a viral infection which resulted in paraplegia (T6 complete). 'My mother took early retirement to care for my child – this was also shared by my mother-in-law when her job permitted. I felt totally useless as a mother, being unable to pick up my daughter and having to watch others attend to her needs as I had once done.'

Monica, whose children were aged 18 months and 3 years old, had a car accident in which her husband was killed and her back broken at T12. Her mother-in-law looked after the children during her eight months of hospitalisation. She wrote: 'I felt I missed a vital part of their lives.'

Molly had two children aged 2 and 4 when she was hospitalised with a spinal tumour 10 years ago. She was away from them for 12 weeks. 'I felt bereft whilst in hospital, because they weren't allowed to visit at all (rules of the neuro-surgical ward). I was also *very* scared that I wouldn't be able to look after them properly when I returned home. To begin with, the 2-year-old didn't recognise me and showed me a photo of "her mummy" (that really broke my heart!).'

Eunice had four children ranging in age from 13 years to 18 months old. She was paralysed as the result of a virus, transverse myelitis, when she was 39 years old in 1964. She wrote: 'At the time I felt divorced from them all as I was in hospital for so long and trying to come to terms with my disability. I grew away from them.'

If the child is very young (under 2 years old) and bonds with the substitute carer, this can cause problems when the mother returns home. Mary's sister had looked after her 15-month-old daughter during her four months in hospital;

when she came home she found that 'Joanne seemed very shy with me and preferred my sister. Joanne never seemed to want me.'

Bridget's daughter, aged 13 months at the time of her accident, established a very strong bond with her father who looked after her during Bridget's five months in hospital. 'When I returned home, I not only had to face the intense jealousy that I felt for their relationship but also my daughter's rage when she was confronted with me rather than her father. I remember the first two mornings that I went in to pick her up from her cot she screamed at me. I felt rejected, guilty, jealous and angry – a misery far worse than I felt at being paralysed.'

Twenty-seven of us had to rely on a number of different arrangements for childcare whilst in hospital and this sometimes caused problems. 'They very much wanted me at home and were disturbed by the variety of carers they had,' wrote Hilary.

Many of us find that, even while lying flat on our backs in hospital, we are the ones who have to organise to keep the family together and cared for. Bridget, for instance, found herself making numerous telephone calls from the spinal unit to arrange care for her daughter.

You won't be able to . . .

Most of us were very nervous about caring for our children once we left hospital. This is not really surprising. After all, before disability, we are unlikely to have any knowledge of how someone in a wheelchair copes with anything – let alone looking after young children. Bridget remembers the sense of shock she felt when the hospital social worker said that she would continue to be her daughter's main carer.

Mary, injured at the level of T12, wrote: 'After my accident my daughter was 1 ½ and I did not think I could cope for some reason – maybe I had had too much time to think. Now, if I'm not breast-feeding Joseph (4 months) or seeing to Thomas (2 ½) in the toilet, I am trying to cook a meal for my husband at work and Joanne and James at school.' And this is the experience of the majority of us; paraplegia does not excuse women from their major caring role within families and tetraplegic women also return to being the main carer of their children but with more practical help.

The physical care of a small child or baby can present practical problems for a mother in a wheelchair, but most of these can be solved. Bathing a baby in the sink is a common solution to bathtime; some mothers have adapted the sides of cots so they can get their child out easily. Jemma wrote: 'When my daugher was very young I wrapped her up in a cocoon so she could be picked up from her cot with one hand. Then I laid her on a pillow on my lap for changing and feeding.'

The physical surroundings to which we return are of paramount importance. It is the inaccessible parts of the home which handicap a paraplegic mother rather than the wheelchair itself. For a tetraplegic woman, having the use of someone else's hands to do what she cannot do herself enables her to look after her children. The tragedy is not paralysis but physical limitations, as well as limitations placed on us by non-disabled people's reactions to our disability.

Julia, who became a tetraplegic as a result of a spinal abscess, found that, unknown to her, her husband was told by her consultant that she would be totally unable to look after herself, let alone her children. Her husband then took the children (aged 2½ and 5½) out of the country and started divorce proceedings. When she applied for custody she found that her consultant would not back her in her determination to look after the children and she now has access to them only during the school holidays. When they come to stay with her, 'I care for them with the help of a live-in au pair, with no problems. Visits out are taken care of by friends or my parents.'

Samantha experienced the same attitude from her consultant, which she felt partly contributed to her husband leaving her 15 months after she returned home. She is completely paralysed from the neck down but when she returned from seven months in hospital, 'I did look after them [her children] myself, with the help of a woman coming in daily and friends.'

The medical profession does seem to have a strange attitude to women's potential and actual capabilities after paralysis. Any independence and return to what we were doing before is seen to be dependent upon a spouse or parent being available to help care for us. As Julia put it, 'He [her consultant] decided that I could not manage because he knew my husband was leaving me, and without a man I would be unable to cope! Who wants to cope with a man who doesn't care and who says a man is a necessity to enable you to manage?'

Bridget's consultant told her, 'I would be quite capable of returning home to look after my 13-month-old daughter . . . until, that is, he found out that I was a single parent living on my own. I was, of course, able to look after my daughter without any help at all, but only because the local authority provided me with a flat which was suitable for someone in a wheelchair. I was then able to return to work and carry on life as a single working mother, but again only because there were certain physical things that made this possible – the building in which I worked was accessible; I could drive and could afford the deposit for a car leased through Motability; the local authority subsidised the cost of a childminder and also provided me with a home help to do my housework. All these things facilitated my return to life as it was before my accident; without them I couldn't have done it.' This again emphasises the lack of physical and material resources as major problems, and it is these things which handicap us, not our disabilities.

Kisses and cuddles

When children are small, the difficulties of physical contact may be particularly heartbreaking for those of us who are tetraplegic. Samantha writes: 'The one thing I missed and found very difficult to cope with, with my sons being still small, was lack of touch, not being able to hug them, bath them and put them to bed.'

The limitations on physical contact can come as a shock to paraplegic women, too. Bridget remembers: 'the sadness I felt at not being able to feel my daughter as she sat on my lap. Other forms of physical contact can compensate, however; I hug my daughter in my arms and forget about the numbness of my legs.' A tetraplegic woman can compensate with kisses and asking her children to stroke her face.

Hilary, whose sons were aged 4 and 6 when she became paralysed, writes, 'The fact that I was in a wheelchair made no difference to the children's attitude to me. I was their mother and that's all that mattered.' And June wrote as a grandmother, 'To my new grandson, I am a wonder gran; I have a chair, and the sides come off, plus four wheels and a lift. I can be pushed around and I don't go flitting about.'

Older children

Older children may present less problems in terms of care arrangements while we are hospitalised but, as they are more aware of what has happened, they can present greater problems in other ways. 'My only son who was 20 years old started college the day of the accident,' wrote Marion. 'He never settled at college and left. The effect on his life has been the greatest.' As mothers we feel guilty about the effect our absence has on our children. Phyllis said: 'I think I let my son down by not being available when he needed me.'

Sometimes these problems are made worse by the circumstances of, and after, the injury. Theresa had three sons aged 6, 7 and 9 when she was hospitalised for a total of 18 months. She was unable to return home to her first and second floor maisonette. Her father died while she was in hospital and her husband was unable to cope. As everything became too much for her mother to deal with, the children eventually went to boarding school. After she came out of hospital it took another 18 months to get accessible accommodation sorted out, by which time her husband had left home. The effect of all this on her children was, she says, 'BAD. Especially the youngest; he had tantrums, violent periods or wanted to jump out of the window. The eldest had to act as a father figure which is probably affecting him now (at 19) as he has become unsettled with his job and home life.' However, Theresa also says, 'They have been marvellous at helping me with shopping, getting my chair out of the car, pushing, etc. I have always tried to go to their school activities, open day, etc. and behave as a normal mother, have friends to stay, etc. and they treat me as an ambulant person and expect me to do everything. And grumble and groan about cleaning their bedrooms and tidying up as most children would do, anyway.'

Paula, who had four-year-old twins and a 13-year-old son, was paralysed after her husband stabbed her. She was in hospital for almost a year. 'It was very traumatic and had a great effect on the children (twins) who became withdrawn, nervous and suffered bed wetting and nightmares. My eldest son ran away from his grandmother, ended up in a children's home and committed a crime – theft. He subsequently committed suicide at 15.' After such a tragic start to her life as a mother with a disability, Paula can now write 'Being a mum in a wheelchair is great. It was not so for me at first because I had a lot of adjusting to do emotionally, and to find out who I really was. As small children (4 onwards) I had a lot of help but since aged about 6 [they are now 10] I have had none. We go everywhere together, swimming, movies, shopping, etc. After all these years I am only now discovering who I am, and what I am capable of doing. I enjoy my independence, making my own decisions and only having myself to answer to. My children are my greatest treasure, but of importance too is the satisfaction that I still have a full and active life – more so than before my injury.'

With older children, those of us who are tetraplegic do not face the practical problems of physical care confronted by tetraplegic mothers of younger children. Georgina, a mother of four sons, aged between 7 and 15 years old when she had her car accident which left her tetraplegic, wrote, 'I feel being a mother and just to be there with them was an advantage as they were at an age when they were very independent children. I feel a mother's advice is just the same, whether able or disabled.' She went on: 'although children can be most exhausting at times, there is no more difficulty, really, coping with them from a wheelchair than otherwise. Coping physically is impossible. Mentally you need to develop a lot of patience. My advice is just don't give up as it always seems to work out right in the end.'

A number of us mentioned how considerate and helpful we found our older children to be. Fiona described the 'astonishing matter-of-fact helpfulness and reliability from my 17- year-old son when I went back to work. He helped with stairs and access four times a day with no fuss at all.'

Wendy's son and daughter were aged 19 and 14 when she became a tetraplegic after falling downstairs at home. Although they found it difficult they obviously played an important role in enabling her to cope. She writes, 'My son found it difficult to cope with the change in our lives but helped me a lot to make the effort to try to resume my life as normally as possible. My daughter became the "Mum" of the family whilst I was away but very quickly allowed me to take over again once I felt able to . . . I found it difficult at first to feel a normal mum in a wheelchair but they wouldn't let me off being a mum again.'

However, sometimes it can take time for older children to adapt, as Janet found. 'My sons (aged 19 and 17) were a long time accepting the fact that I had changed from a very active mother to someone who had to ask for practically everything.'

A long period in hospital for their mother can leave children fearing a repetition of the separation. 'My son even now does not like me going away or into hospital,' wrote Hannah. 'For ages after I returned home they [her children] didn't like travelling on the road that they travelled to the hospital to visit me.' And a few women felt that their injuries had had long-lasting and devastating effects on their children. Daisy wrote: 'The younger child (aged 6 at the time) never recovered; he is now 39 and still will not discuss it.'

Having a child after injury

Twenty of us have had children following paralysis (and three were pregnant when injured). For most of us this has been a positive experience, and we have emphasised what is possible rather than the limitations experienced.

Most women did not consult any medical opinion before conceiving a child, and 13 had no problems with their labour and delivery. 'There were no problems,' wrote Kathy. 'The first I had a forceps delivery. The second I had a natural birth. The first I did not feel anything and the doctor did it for me (forceps delivery – 48 stitches). He was 5lb 13 ozs.The second I felt everything and the doctor was there but only said push and I did a natural birth, no stitches and she was 8lb 4 oz.'

Karen was 4½ months pregnant at the time of her accident and injury, and wrote, 'The casualty hospital left me alone in an X-ray room with the X-rays of my broken bones hanging up so I could read them! That was how I learnt I had broken my back, though I didn't let them know I knew. I was pregnant and terrified.' She had an uncomfortable pregnancy as she spent the next three months on her back. 'I was naturally worried as to whether my baby would be normal after such a jolt. The birth was in a maternity hospital, though they could have coped at the spinal unit. It was an induced labour, high forceps delivery and very carefully monitored. My husband was present for the delivery. My daughter was 'light for dates' and dysmature [the placenta had stoped growing], weighing 5½ lbs. She had breathing problems and was in intensive paediatric care for two weeks.'

Karen faced the difficult choice of either looking after her infant daughter or staying in the spinal unit to learn to do all the things that she would need to do once she was home. 'I made the decision to send my baby home from the spinal unit so I could get home too. She was looked after by a qualified nanny and my husband. I missed her terribly but I suspect I made the right decision. It was important that I got back home as quickly as possible and start leading a normal family life.' The decision was obviously the right one, for she is now able to write. 'There are no problems to being a good mother in a wheelchair.'

Helen was eight weeks pregnant when a viral infection left her paralysed (T6 complete). She already had a 13-month-old daughter. 'When I returned home I was 20 weeks pregnant with my second child and facing the full horror of my new physical condition.' Her child was born brain damaged by the virus which had paralysed her and only lived five days. It took her and her husband another two years to make the decision to have another child. They consulted a genetic counsellor who said there should be no problems. 'As I had no periods following paralysis several courses of Clomid [fertility drug] were necessary to achieve a pregnancy.' She had a difficult pregnancy but the Caesarian delivery went very smoothly. 'All the doctors and nurses were very excited at the safe arrival of our second daughter.'

Medical opinion is that usually pregnancy for a paraplegic woman should go smoothly; there are no extra risks involved to the baby as long as care is taken to find out when a woman goes into labour as if you are paraplegic you may not be aware when this happens. However, there are risks attached to pregnancy and labour for a tetraplegic woman, and tragically for Eva (whose level of paralysis is C5 incomplete) medical advice and treatment were inadequate. Although she was told (inaccurately) 'that there were no special problems related to quadraplegics during pregnancy and labour', she had high blood pressure and fits during both her labours. Both children were born severely handicapped (although it is not clear whether this is a result of her own disability) and she has had a very difficult time looking after them. 'My son has hydrocephaly [a congenital malformation] and can make no progress in growing up. I cannot manage him at all now he is too big for me to hold. It takes one full-time and another part-time helper to care for him, and it is still a struggle. My daughter is severely mentally and physically retarded and it is doubtful whether she can see. She is therefore also heavy and difficult for me to handle. I still feed her myself, which is one less problem, but with these two I have not really begun to even think about being a mother in a wheelchair yet, more just getting on with it!' Her medical advisers are still not able to tell her why this has happened. 'They are not sure if the children were affected by a poor blood supply to the uterus, nor is it definite that the fits were attributable to tetraplegia or not. They were not normal eclamptic fits [caused by high blood pressure].'

Tetraplegic women do successfully deliver normal babies, but there are risks involved which require close monitoring and prompt treatment. In fact, of the four tetra-plegic women who answered the questionnaire who have had children since paralysis, Eva was the only one who experienced any problems. Fran, whose level of injury is C6/7 (incomplete), had twins 'and managed to bring them up without any help'. Her biggest problem seems to have been having a husband 'who always said "You can't do that in a wheelchair". Two years ago I divorced my husband and since then I have learned to drive and learned to live again (nothing is impossible).' Her labour was normal – except that it was only when she was in labour that twins were detected. She had a forceps delivery. She wrote: 'I would have had no problems at all if I had had one, but being two I did have help with the feeding, for the first six months. I bathed them in the kitchen sink and lifted them out on to a changing mat on the draining boards. Nappies, toiletries and pins were kept on a dinner trolley, so they were all at hand and could be easily moved from room to room.'

Although some paraplegic and tetraplegic women have painless labours, this depends on the level of injury and how complete the lesion is. Mary (T12/L1), who has had three children since paralysis, wrote, 'My labours were very pain-fully normal.'

Where there are problems during pregnancy, they mostly stem from the greater risk of pressure sores, the difficulties of transferring from, and generally moving about in, a wheelchair in the later months of pregnancy. When delivery involves an episiotomy [a small cut made at the bottom of the vagina at the moment of delivery], care has to be taken to prevent the stitched wound from turning into a pressure sore. However, bedrest or sitting on a cushion with the centre scooped out can stop this happening.

Those of us who have had children since our disablement worried about how we would cope with the physical care of a new baby. But as Kathy, mother of two (and intending to have more), put it, 'I had no real problems; the only big one was how to carry the new baby so I used a tie on baby carrier that wraps around yourself. I have no help at all. My husband works like anyone else and I cope on my own. Don't be afraid to have children. They are wonderful.' She also childminds an 18-month-old and a 6-year-old child.

Keeping children safe

One of the most worrying aspects of childcare for disabled mothers is how to keep our children safe when we cannot run quickly to rescue them from danger. Bridget wrote: 'While my daughter is young (she's 4 now) I won't go anywhere which is unfamiliar and may contain potential dangers unless I take another adult with me. However, where I know the dangers – within my home, in the streets that I am familiar with, in the park, etc. – I am confident about looking after her. When you can't physically restrain your child you learn other methods of control – which I personally believe is better for you and the child, anyway.'

Molly wrote: 'My greatest problem was chasing after them if they went near the road/canal/strange dog, etc. I developed a very loud and authoritative voice-tone.' She went on, 'The toddler stage was very difficult as I couldn't run after them when they were in danger. I shouted! They became very obedient and rarely disobeyed me.'

Karen writes: 'I used a playpen for safety; my daughter and I are very close and "no" has always meant that. I made sure that right from the start she had every encouragement to be independent and think for herself. A child is often removed from a precarious situation before it has had a chance to think it out alone.'

'I wish I had a wheelchair, Mummy'

Many of us worry that we won't be able to do all sorts of things that our children will want us to do. Some of us expressed regret about what we couldn't do, but also satisfaction and joy at what we could do.

Georgina, a tetraplegic, asked her four sons, now grown up but aged 7, 10, 12 and 15 at the time of her accident, whether they felt they had any problems because of her paralysis. They felt there had been 'none whatsoever, except on reflection the youngest felt he missed out on going on as many family outings as perhaps other families. The only disadvantage they feel was having to help with dishes!'

Shirley also felt that her 'youngest child suffered most in that I don't take him here, there and everywhere as I did when his brothers were of a similar age'. Having said that, she then goes on to say that this 8-year-old doesn't seem to be at all bothered by her being in a wheelchair – 'he uses it as a climbing frame'. Those of us with young children often find that they think it a great adventure to ride on our laps going down the street. 'It never ceases to amaze me what a different perspective children can have from adults,' wrote Bridget. 'My daughter once sighed as I was putting the bags of shopping on the back of my wheelchair and said, with great feeling, "I wish *I* had a wheelchair, Mummy"!'

Mothers in wheelchairs have an important contribution to make, as demonstrated by Molly who has two children. 'We lived in a rural area with few facilities. I and two friends started playgroups in our own houses and then one in a local community centre. I always took a full role in this and took my turn looking after everyone else's children, too. Hard work but rewarding. I was always a captive audience, though, and children loved me to read to them (for hours!). Maybe I had more time for them than busy mums who are always doing housework!' She went on, 'When they went to school, I used to go into school, too, one afternoon, to help with small groups of children – reading or baking, etc. I wanted all their friends to be used to

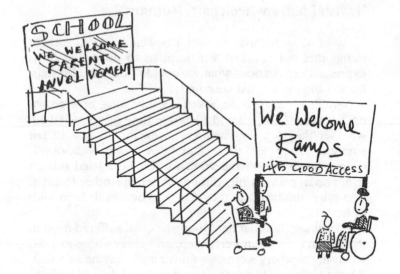

seeing me in a wheelchair so I wouldn't be thought of as a freak. Now they're at comprehensive, I still go to all school functions so that I am known to all their friends and teachers. As far as I know, my children have never been ashamed or embarrassed by me, and other children have accepted me as I am. I always refuse to keep a low profile at home. It's paid off, I think.'

However, some of us did express a lot of regret that activities with our children were restricted. 'We do not go out as much as before,' wrote Jane, a mother of three children aged 4, 8 and 12. Emily worried that her children might resent the fact that she is in a wheelchair and commented, 'I miss the trips, social arrangements and sporting activities previously enjoyed.'

Hilary also wrote, 'It was sad not to be able to take them to the zoo or out shopping or for walks.' This handicap is a direct result of the lack of resources which would enable her to engage in these activities with her children. Access to public buildings, toilet facilities, parking facilities, availability of people to help when needed, electric outdoor wheelchairs when required – all these are items which can and should be provided. Many of us do, of course, find that we are able to do all the things with our children that a non-disabled mother can do, but this is because the physical obstacles have been removed. For example, access to schools is often a problem for mothers of school-age children. Yet Elsa reports how her son's school has been very helpful and co-operative and has provided ramps to enable her to get into the school and be as involved in school activities as any other mother. This is how it should be for all of us.

Celia, who walks with crutches, commented, 'Being a "mother on crutches" brings problems and frustrations, i.e. unable to carry a child, hold his hand whilst walking, come to his aid easily and quickly.' Her son was 8½ months old when she was injured. Now he is 22 and she says, 'I recently asked him what effect it had on him and he told me he cannot remember even thinking about it . . . Broadly, young children accept their parents as part of their lives, whatever they are. Obviously, as my son grew older there were moments when he wished I could play, run, etc. with him. But unfulfilled wishes about parents are common, in some form or another, to all children.'

9.

Growing Older

Almost everyone fears getting older because we associate frailty, loss of independence and illness with old age. As disabled women we often feel we have more to fear. Yet the experience of those who are already in their 60s and 70s seems to a large extent to contradict these apprehensions. Some do experience additional problems of pain and greater restrictions on mobility but on the whole it seems that old age, like most other stages of the life cycle, is much the same for us as for our non-disabled sisters. Thirty-eight women who took part in this project are over 60; 89 are between the ages of 40 and 59. This chapter is about our feelings in relation to the idea of getting older and also to the actual experience.

Looking to the future

Many of us are fearful of the prospect of getting older. Our lives when young are made possible by the strength in our arms and/or our carers. Those of us in our 20s, 30s and 40s fear that growing older will mean the loss of these vital strengths. Nadia, recently injured at the age of 24, writes, 'I am worried about how I will cope when I am older as strength will begin to go.' And Erica says, 'Old age scares me a bit as I know how much I rely on my husband's strength to provide my freedom of activity . . . ' For Wendy, also, it is the prospect of anything happening to her husband which is the worst aspect of growing older as she fears that if anything did happen she would have to go into residential care.

Some of us who do not have husbands or partners fear that independent living will become impossible as we grow older. Julia, who recently became a tetraplegic and whose husband left taking the children with him, writes, 'The thought terrifies me as the day approaches when I will be totally dependent on someone else. I just hope there is someone there when it arrives.' Often our worries are related to whether we will have sufficient money to pay for whatever care we might need if we should have greater personal care needs when we get older. Compensation or an adequate pension can make all the difference to how we view the future. For example, Bridget, a single parent who successfully sued for compensation following her accident, is confident she will have sufficient income to pay for personal care in her own home should this become necessary.

Libby has particular fears as an incomplete tetraplegic, currently able to walk but with weak hands and arms. 'I worry a lot that, as I grow older, I will get weaker and have to use a wheelchair which would mean an end to independence, my arms being too weak for me to push myself around in the street, for instance.'

Many of us are particularly worried about the prospect of a loss of independence implying residential care. Gina, a tetraplegic with a high level of independence in her daily life at the moment, writes, 'I feel it's rather daunting getting older. I need every muscle that I have now to manage with some degree of independence. As things slow down and weaken, it will obviously be very hard. I have a horror of being in a home and not being able to organise my life as I do now.'

Anita, who spent 10 years in residential care before she achieved independent living for herself and her husband (both of them tetraplegic), says of the prospect of getting older, 'I don't like the idea at all.' She continues: 'It is hard for most people to envisage growing older in a society that cares very little for its elderly population. If I was a fit able woman, I don't think it would have worried me so much, but the growing dependency I will have on other people is very frightening. Mentally, I cannot cope with the idea of getting frail and going into any institution. If I had no responsibility to loved ones, I would take the coward's way out and take a correct overdose. I could not suffer the indignities of institutional care again; once was enough.'

Molly fears that her paralysis may increase as she grows older. Now aged 38, her paralysis started when she was a schoolgirl as a result of a tumour. She writes: 'I'm terrified that my arms will become paralysed, too [if the tumour grows]. My main fear is that I won't be able to get to the toilet or keep myself clean. I'm afraid of being dependent and losing my dignity and self-respect.' Such loss of independence is, of course, experienced by many people as they grow old, but perhaps our disability means we have a greater perception of how we will feel about it when it happens.

Some of us assume that our paralysis inevitably means we have a shorter life expectancy. Martha writes: 'I don't imagine I'll live to be very old,' and Katherine, disabled 10 years ago, says, 'The older I get the sadder I feel and the longer I've been disabled I think I won't see my children grow up. I have a great fear of death. I like my life really, but I know paraplegics don't live to a great old age.' She is not actually right about this. Up until the Second World War, many paraplegics and tetraplegics died of paralysis-associated complications (primarily kidney failure) because of a failure to recognise the appropriate practical and medical responses. Now, however, paraplegics and tetraplegics are living into their 60s, 70s and 80s.

Moreover, the actual experience of growing older seems to be more positive and less daunting than the fears we have as young women contemplating getting older. It is interesting that the younger women who filled in our questionnaire often had more to say about their fears of growing older than the older women had to say about actual problems they were facing. Some of us who are 60 and over had little to say about the experience, other than advice about the importance of diet, exercise and posture. Elspeth, injured in 1958 and now aged 73, did not comment on her feelings about getting older but offered the following advice, which has obviously kept her healthy and active. 'Cut down on fat, salt and sugar. Avoid convenience foods with their deadly additives. Have one properly cooked meal each day – meat or fish with green vegetables as fresh as possible. Grill rather than fry. Coping in a wheelchair is quite an exercise. Keep your spine as erect, and your back as straight, as possible.'

Some of the older women who did write of the restrictions and aches and pains associated with getting older also, however, expressed their belief that their experiences were no different from those of their non-disabled friends. Margot, aged 70 and paralysed for 30 years, wrote, 'It's tougher and I'm slower and get tired quicker and haven't so much energy or stamina. I feel as if I'm gradually grinding to a halt, but no more than my able-bodied friends of the same age.' Her major worry at the moment is in fact her husband's health, as he has been hospitalised for some time and her life to a large extent revolves around visiting him. 'Life would have been very different if he had been well – I don't think he realises I'm disabled!'

Daisy was the only over-70-year-old who expressed fears about growing older. Paralysed from the waist in 1952 and now aged 74, her experience of a broken leg a year ago has contributed to her anxiety. 'I dread very much getting any older and I wonder how much longer I shall be able to go on being totally independent.' Living on her own, it is only within the last year that she has had help with her housework and with changing her catheter.

Perhaps a final word on the *prospect* of old age should go to Jocelyn. Aged 42 and injured in a fall from a horse 26 years ago, she changed her career from horse-riding to training dogs, married and had two sons. Her response to the question on old age was 'Old age? I've never given it any thought at all.'

Growing older

What about the actual experience of getting older? The

following sections of this chapter cover some of the experiences of aging which women focused on. In writing about
growing older, we identified not only the issue of aging but
also what it is like spending many years with paralysis. Some
women in their 40s and 50s who had been paralysed for
many years wrote of the experience of paralysis in terms of
growing older; other women in their 60s and 70s thought
that growing older would not bring about problems until
they were in their 80s. As Edith, a 70-year-old tetraplegic,
said, 'Everything is easier now I am older. The problem will
be when I am really old.'

Hard work

Many of us find that, as we grow older, we are finding it hard
work being in a wheelchair or on crutches. Most people tire
more quickly as they get older, but for us the problem is
more acute as we have to put more energy just into daily living. As the years of disability pass, these greater efforts can
affect how we feel about growing older. Alison now aged 50
and paralysed 22 years ago, admits 'how run down one gets
as an older paraplegic'. And Eunice, aged 62 and paralysed
for 23 years, finds that 'the daily chores get more tiring'. Liz
warns: 'The difficulty of looking after yourself in the long-
term is that you can turn your daily life into something
resembling an assault course.'

Cynthia, who was until very recently in full-time employment as a teacher, found that, 'it was not hard at first to cope
with, but now at 59, after 27 years of paraplegia as well as a
busy professional and family life, I am finding things hard
going.' She advises: 'don't get over tired and allow extra
time to do everything.' Sarah would agree: 'lead an active
life, but unless you have the ambition to be an Olympic
champion, don't overstrain the limbs you are still able to
use, for over a lifetime they are going to be under constant
pressure.'

It is worrying that the aging process itself will result in
health problems which may be more difficult for us to

handle because of paralysis. As Celia says, 'Growing older is something that all women must come to terms with, disabled or not. But I do worry that other problems of aging will loom and cause trouble. I also sometimes find it hard to imagine myself as an old disabled person. I sometimes do not accept this disability is forever.'

Janet, now aged 62, writes of her experiences of 24 years as a paraplegic, which include health problems experienced by many able-bodied women. For example, she had a mastectomy six years ago, and this must have contributed to the physical difficulties of living with paralysis. 'I am much slower now, after 24 years,' she writes. 'I get colds easier and find it more difficult to transfer from my wheelchair to other places. However,' she continues, 'taking a look at my life in a chair, over the years, I find it has not been so bad. I have had more good moments than bad; keeping a sense of humour is essential. Learning to laugh at one's predicament helps enormously.'

Menopause

The menopause for some causes problems; for others it is, as Fiona says, 'quite a treat!' Valerie writes: 'I feel more at ease with myself now I have got over the worst effects of the menopause . . . I experienced a lot of emotional disturbance and lack of confidence, but from talking to my able-bodied friends they seem to suffer far worse symptoms and complications. Just talking to other women going through it has helped me. We aren't really any different.'

For someone like Jean, a tetraplegic, who regrets the indignity of asking her husband to change sanitary pads, the end of the menopause is a relief. If the menopause brings with it heavier and more frequent periods this can at best be inconvenient and at worst extremely distressing for a wheelchair user because of the practical difficulties. Nadine contemplated the menopause with anxiety: 'I am very apprehensive about the menopause. It may be difficult to cope with heavy menstruation. Ordinary periods are bad enough.'

Sometimes a hysterectomy brings a troublesome meno-pause to an end, as Hazel writes, 'The menopause was a ter-rible problem. For years I'd had very heavy periods which became continual. Then I had a hysterectomy and I've never looked back since, never felt better!' However, the menopause does not always cause problems. For instance, Mavis experienced only 'minor problems which I coped with quite well'.

Cynthia found that the greatest difficulty while going through the menopause was getting too tired, which may have been aggravated by the greater efforts required to get through daily life in a wheelchair. 'My worst problem,' she wrote, 'was not being able to cope when I was tired – I fre-quently burst into tears. I should always have allowed lots of extra time to do everything as rushing about had a terrible effect. I realise now that I must have been awful to live with and it was mostly to do with that feeling of not being able to cope.'

Blanche wrote of the physical and emotional problems brought about by the menopause and how she tackled them. 'One particular problem with the menopause was a build up of fluid in the tissue which led to sores if the tem-perature changed, and there was some friction on my skin. I now always wear Tubigrip circular bandages instead of socks. I had bouts of nostalgia, a flurry of sexual activity and a determination to break out of my work and ritual depen-dencies; you could call it discontent! Or another attack of delayed adolescence! I learned to relax some of the rigid spinal unit training and felt much better for it. Why should a paraplegic who is no good at games have to show everyone they can work twice as hard as an average person? A bit of self-indulgence can make one feel much more kindly dis-posed to the world in general.'

'Life sentence?'

Twenty-seven of us had been paralysed for more than 25 years, 10 for more than 30 years, and some of these women felt this had been going on for far too long. Eva wrote: 'I'm fed up with being disabled. I feel it has gone on long enough.' And her feelings are shared by many of us who were paralysed when still children or in our teens or early 20s. For Annie, injured when aged 18 and now 27, her fears of growing older are bound up with her regrets at what she has lost. 'I fear that I might feel even more depressed looking back and realising all the things I couldn't do and missed . . .'

Yet Marsha, paralysed nine years ago when she was 55 years old, says, 'The longer you are paralysed, the more you come to terms with it. At 64 I feel fit.' She took on a new lease of life after her husband died. 'When he died I was left to take over all the household problems, whereas before he had done it all and I had felt inferior. He treated me as though I wasn't able to cope even where I could. I am now enjoying every minute of it. I feel more happy and contented than I have felt in a long time.'

Sometimes, although years of disability are exhausting, things are still not as bad as we had previously feared. Beth, now aged 45 and paralysed when she was 14, writes, 'It was easier to feel normal when young because I had far more energy and was less unattractive. I feel that 30 years of coping with paraplegia and a demanding full-time job have exhausted me. On the other hand, I am fairly fit and far more healthy at 45 than I would have thought possible 30 years ago when first paralysed. My fears then of constant hospitalisation or not being able to lead an independent life have been proved unfounded.'

If our general experience of paralysis is very negative it is not surprising that the prospect of growing older, of spending more and more years with increasing restrictions and pain, fills us with dread. Kitty, who has acute and permanent pain as well as other problems, says, 'I don't want to live to be old as a paralysed woman.' This pessimism is echoed by Ellen, aged 50, who says, 'My feelings about growing old are: I hope I don't live to see tomorrow. As a failed paraplegic I don't feel qualified to give any advice.' Her paralysis in a road accident was followed by divorce three months after she came out of hospital and her father's death. She was unable to go back to her previous job. From having a full and enjoyable life, she felt that spinal cord injury had deprived her of everything.

Conclusion

The prospect of growing older as a disabled woman may seem daunting, yet from the experience of those women in their 60s and 70s it is difficult to state categorically that disability necessarily implies greater problems in old age.

Indeed, many older women felt there were positive advantages in growing older, in particular the fact that their friends and relatives were also growing older and slowing down. Edith, now 71 and paralysed since she was 40, declared, 'Now I am older everything is much easier. There are no children to be cared for. My husband is as disabled as I am. Relatives and friends have all slowed down. No one expects an old lady to look glamorous. Age has great compensations for me.'

Margery identified another advantage of growing older when she wrote, 'I have seen great changes in public awareness, equipment and financial provision in my 24 years of disability – though there is a long way still to go. On the whole,' she concludes, 'I think we must all make the best of our lives and accept what we cannot change. This certainly becomes easier as we get older.'

Samantha also identified that, in growing older, disability becomes easier for her to cope with. Once the adjustment to disability has been made, she says, 'Life can only get better.' She goes on, 'Time is a great factor and it feels really good when you no longer look at people walking down the street and wish it was you.' Lorna writes that 'I feel less bothered about growing older as a paralysed woman than my more vanity-conscious able-bodied friends. They often say I am far more at peace with life than they are.'

As paraplegics and tetraplegics, in growing older, we may experience some loss of independence, as we may no longer be able to keep up the considerable effort of 'the daily assault course', and we may lose the help of those on whom we had depended. We may have increased pain, develop arthritis and other health problems. However, it is important to recognise that some of the problems mentioned in this chapter apply to all people growing older and cannot be directly attributed to spinal cord injury. Deborah says 'I think there are some problems like getting fatter and slower and losing track of one's friends that cannot be blamed on the paraplegia, and we are in danger of doing so.'

10.

Incontinence

Bladders

'I think that my bladder is the worst thing, even than being in a wheelchair.' Theresa speaks for most of us who feel that, while bowel incontinence does not usually cause major problems, our lives are made miserable and severely limited by having to cope with incontinent bladders.

When the spinal cord is damaged, feeling of, and/or control over our bladder and bowels is affected. If we cannot feel when we need to pee or empty the bowels there may be the ever present worry of either happening unexpectedly. Imagine being at a party and a puddle suddenly appearing under your wheelchair. Or sitting on someone's beautiful new sofa and realising that you have just peed all over it. Or accepting a lift in someone's car and worrying all the way home that when you get out there may be a tell-tale wet patch on the seat. And how can you enjoy making love when you're worried all the time that you might pee on your partner?

Incontinence is humiliating. It can place a far greater limitation on our lives than being in a wheelchair or using crutches. Yet it is very rarely spoken about or confronted as an issue.

There are a number of ways of dealing with incontinence, all of which have disadvantages. The clearest message from our collective experiences is that each person is different and that what works for one will not for another. We each have to sort out a solution which best suits our body and life style. Unfortunately, our experience of the medical profession is often that its members have set ideas about how to deal with incontinence and attempt to impose particular regimes and techniques on everyone, disregarding individual needs and differences.

Bladder training

There is a marked contrast in the experiences of the 99 women who use bladder training and those who use some other method. Bladder training means that you literally train your bladder to respond to a sensation and/or movement. The most common method taught at spinal units is to tap the abdomen, but women also use a variety of other methods, such as straining or bending double. In theory, bladder training deals with incontinence by accustoming the bladder to be 'expressed' in this way every four hours or so. In practice, most of us find we have to empty our bladders far more often; that certain foods or drinks, or the menstrual cycle, will affect our control; that we may have difficulty in emptying the bladder completely. Persistent bladder infections (sometimes called urinary tract infections or cystitis) are also an occupational hazard for spinal cord injured people.

Most of us who use bladder training feel we can never forget our bladders. 'It dominates 99.9 per cent of my time,' wrote Katherine. The effectiveness of this method depends on being able to keep to a strict timetable of input and output. It is possible to be in reasonable control of this at home where we can get to a loo when we need to, but even there, as Deborah says, 'It's the time and effort it takes to cope with this that dominates my life. Bladder training at best only gives me three hours between toilet visits. Compared to a lot of people this is good.' And it is. Phyllis has to express her bladder 'nearly every hour'. Each visit is not just a matter of seconds, either. As Fran points out, 'I can be on the toilet half an hour or longer.' For many these visits carry on all night, too. Abigail writes: 'I get up a minimum of four times nightly, very often more.'

However, it is outside the home that bladder training exerts its real toll and dominates every activity. As Hilary says, 'incontinence controls the whole programming of my working and social life.' And Christine commented, 'Every drink has to be planned in a busy college/school day.' Emily, a secondary school teacher has abandoned bladder training in despair because 'It prevents *living*, let alone working'. It involves a constant juggling of decisions and plans, as Theresa illustrates. 'It's the old story of: Dare I have a coffee now? What time am I going out? I'll have to leave an hour or so between drinking and going to the loo before going out. How much dare I drink when out socially before I need the loo? Or, I can't have a drink during the evening when I'm out as I won't want to sit on a wet pad.'

So many of our experiences illustrate the limitations set on all paraplegic and tetraplegic women's lives by the lack of accessible toilets, especially for those who use bladder training. 'If I go anywhere I try to find out if the loos are accessible. If they are not, I won't go,' says Phyllis. And Katherine writes, 'I'm OK in my own home but hopeless anywhere else. If there's no accessible loo, we can't be long or else I just get soaked and irritable. Visiting friends we drive miles to find the nearest town with a disabled loo before we get there. I don't stay at friends' houses. All our friends come here to visit.' Liz concludes: 'Its capacity to blight your pleasure while out or travelling is considerable and this has never really changed.'

The longest time anyone reported they could leave between visits to the lavatory was five hours, but the average was every two hours, depending on other factors. 'If I go to the lavatory every two hours (at the most) I can stay dry, as long as I don't drink too much – then it's only an hour I can last out,' says Molly. The effect of all this on our lives does not seem to be taken into account when the medical profession insists that, for most of us, bladder training is the best option.

It is the women who can't properly empty their bladder who have a particularly difficult time. Shirley writes: 'I can partially empty my bladder but *still* go in between trips to the loo.' Liz offered this advice. 'In the early days no one told me to express my bladder again after the first release of urine, thus I was often wet an hour or so later. By expressing at least twice, sometimes three times, every time I go to the loo I can avoid being wet for long periods.'

The amount of warning – when there is any warning – of the need to go to the loo is usually very short. Christine says: 'I know when I want to go with approximately 8–10 seconds warning. So I either have to be near a loo or go before I need to and/or control my drinking so I don't need to.' One of the disadvantages of being able to walk with calipers is illustrated by Leila who gets what many wheelchair users would regard as a wonderful amount of warning, and yet finds bladder training 'totally ineffective! I've got 2–5 minutes to get to a toilet and when you're walking that's not a long time.'

Some of us have sensation when the bladder is full and so bladder training can be really effective. For instance, Jane says: 'I can now tell when my bladder is full, though not when it is empty. I now empty my bladder when it feels full and also before I go out or to bed, and often before I sit down to a meal. It works very well. I use my abdominal muscles and lean as far forward on the toilet as I can. I can last about four hours between each bladder emptying and normally get up once during the night.' But most of us have to rely on getting to know how our body is likely to work. 'I have just got to know when I'm likely to need to go and how much I can drink and when without getting into difficulties. I manage very well on the whole,' writes Tessa.

Twenty-two of the 99 women using bladder training are tetraplegic. Elaine, who is C6/7 incomplete, used to have a catheter, but had to rely on the district nurse to change it, etc. 'which was a real drag'. So she switched to bladder training, although she has a tough time. 'My bladder does exactly as it wants so I wear home-made incontinence pads. My trousers are often wet but not too bad.' Eileen, injured at C5/6 complete, thinks that bladder training is a joke: 'I just use thick home-made pads and go to the loo four times a day – always wet. I tried to go to the loo "on warning" but never made it in time.'

Although some women find that, in time, they can train

their bladders into reasonable regimes, many others find
that bladder training as a method of incontinence management restricts their lives considerably. It is unfortunate that
the medical and nursing professions are so sold on the idea
of bladder training. The notion of it being the most 'natural'
way to deal with incontinence appears to obscure the enormous disadvantages, as Bridget found when, following her
insistence that she wished to practise self-catheterisation, a
nurse at her spinal unit expressed disgust and regret at such a
solution to the problem.

It is not surprising that women who have changed from
bladder training to some other method expressed an enormous sense of relief and freedom. A total of 59 women had
given up bladder training. However, the alternatives also
have their drawbacks, whether the greater dangers of infections from catheterisation or the traumas of a major operation required for urinary diversions and radio-controlled
implants. The majority of us do in fact put up with bladder
training, though the price we have to pay in terms of
anxiety, embarrassment, planning, time, effort and cur-
tailment of our social and working life can be enormous.

Catheters
A catheter is a thin tube which is inserted into the urethra
(through which urine passes from the bladder and the opening to which is just in front of the vagina).

Indwelling catheters
An indwelling catheter merely means that it is kept in place
for a period of time and that urine drains from the tube into a
bag which is normally strapped to the leg. 'It's like a weight
that's been lifted.' Elspeth expresses the majority opinion
about using an indwelling catheter – that there are some problems but also an overwhelming sense of relief. 'At times I have
considerable leakage with a catheter, usually due to infection.
Otherwise, it's a great relief to be free of the slavery of two-
hourly lifting, hours spent cutting up rolls of cotton wool, etc.
making pads, coping with wet ones and cushion covers.'

A number of the 63 women now using an indwelling catheter had tried other methods first. These trials had often produced considerable frustration and misery, so that the change to a catheter induced a great sense of freedom. Geraldine wrote: 'I tried bladder training for two years but I found that I had to revolve my life around a toilet. When I changed to a catheter it was like someone had unlocked the ball and (toilet!) chain I was tied to.'

Almost all of us have an indwelling catheter inserted during the first days and weeks of paralysis when we are confined to a hospital bed. Becoming free of the catheter and its embarrassing drainage bag, which our visitors try to avoid looking at as it lurks under the bed, is often the first thing we aim for in the early stages of 'rehabilitation'. Not surprisingly, therefore, most of us are very reluctant to change back to an indwelling catheter, and most have done so only out of medical or practical necessity.

Lorna, for instance, had a deterioration in her medical condition which necessitated the continual use of a catheter. 'When the consultant mentioned an indwelling catheter I was very upset at the time, but now I'm glad. It saves me all the worry and gives me much more time in each day.' She has had no problems at all with her catheter and finds it very effective. Julia was paralysed in 1983 as the result of a spinal abscess – 'I did try bladder training but my efforts were unsuccessful. Then I tried self-catheterisation, but this was also unsuccessful due to very strong leg spasms. It was a relief to stay with the indwelling catheter.'

A few of us had tried no method other than a catheter. Helen was eight weeks pregnant at the time of her injury, and had to remain with an indwelling catheter at least until after the baby was born. But when her doctor then tried to persuade her to change to intermittent catheterisation she refused 'as I have had few problems with the indwelling catheter and with two young children I haven't got the time for experimentation'.

The main problems which recurred for those of us who use indwelling catheters were the following: blockages of the catheter caused by sediment in the urine; problems of by-passing [urine leaking out directly from the urethra rather than through the catheter]; bladder stones [caused by a build-up of calcium]; and bladder infections. For some, these problems certainly negated, or at least limited, the lack of worry which is otherwise experienced with an indwelling catheter.

Willa, who was paralysed at L5/S1 in 1966 when she was knocked down by a car, finds that, apart from infections, bladder stones are her problem. Her incontinence 'does dominate' her life 'but I try to ignore it – I *think* I have it under control at the moment'. Naomi found that initially her catheter was often being by-passed and needed changing about every two weeks but that it has been 'much more reliable over the last 12 months. I have been on antibiotics for nine months for abscesses and during this time the catheter was very reliable. Now I have to make sure I drink a lot (which is a bit awkward when going out for the day) to keep it flushed through.'

Geraldine's comment was echoed by a number of us. 'I find using a catheter reasonable but I do get a great deal of soreness from it.' The spiral of difficulties that can occur was described by Mavis who has always used an indwelling catheter since she was paralysed 10 years ago. 'I have inflammation in the urinary tract and my bladder has shrunk, making catheter changes very painful at the change and for long periods afterwards (two to three days).'

'I would like to see a better catheter bag suitable for a woman' – Willa's mild request echoes a general distress about the unattractiveness of an indwelling catheter. Julia commented: 'I wish the leg bags weren't so obvious so that I could maybe wear a skirt or tighter trousers.'

Apart from its unattractiveness, many women had other complaints about the equipment available. Amanda has found 'I am allergic to many catheters and am still trying to get a supply of suitable catheters as the manufacturer has stopped making the only ones I have found suitable. I find this very worrying.'

Nearly everyone who uses a catheter needs help in changing it (which has to be done at intervals which can vary between every few days to weeks), whether she is a paraplegic or tetraplegic. For Helen this is done 'by my husband or district nurse'. She can tell when it needs to be changed. Elsa finds that she can 'change the catheter myself, but I need ancillary help. I get blocked fairly frequently and "by pass". With any block I need to call out a care attendant to help me.'

However, there are some catheters which decide to change themselves and that leads to the embarrassment we all dread, as Julia describes: 'The only problem which arises is if it gets pulled out without me realising, then we end up with puddles everywhere.'

Supra-pubic catheters

Two women use a supra-pubic catheter. This is when the catheter is introduced through the abdominal wall directly into the bladder, rather than through the urethra. Vicky, who uses this method, makes a plea for 'each case to be looked at separately. I had all sorts of problems following admission to a spinal unit for other reasons. They tried to change my routine to fit the standard, with disastrous results. I now have a supra-pubic catheter and it's great – so easy to change by myself. The catheter and leg-bag suit my life style. After my urethra was messed up the change to a supra-pubic catheter was pretty traumatic but all has settled down and I prefer it now.'

Intermittent self-catheterisation

This method of passing urine involves inserting a small catheter each time you need to pee. Sixteen women used this method. The advantages are that it is quick and the bladder can be completely emptied. It is also a procedure which can be done anywhere – if an accessible toilet is not available you can pee into a bottle while sitting in the wheelchair. The disadvantages are that some who use this method also experience quite frequent bladder infections. Emily, for example, had only been using intermittent catheterisation for two months and found that she constantly had bladder infections.

Bridget, however, has found the method suits her perfectly. 'Once I left the spinal unit I stopped bothering about sterile conditions, and in fact re-use catheters which are only supposed to be used once. I wash them under the tap. I have never had a bladder infection since being paralysed four years ago. I think this may have something to do with having successfully prevented the cystitis that I used to get in my late teens and early 20s before I was paralysed. Having got to the stage then of being on antibiotics every three months or so, I read a book called *Understanding Cystitis* by Angela Kilmartin. I stopped taking antibiotics and – by following certain advice such as no coffee or spirits, making sure I completely emptied my bladder (I had a tendency to urine retention even before I was paralysed owing to a very strong sphincter – intermittent catheterisation, of course, overcomes this problem completely!), etc. – I kept myself completely free of cystitis for years before my accident. I think my body has built up its own resistance to bacteria in my bladder because I didn't rely on antibiotics and now this means that I don't get infections even following paralysis.'

Implants
Artificial implants to operate the bladder are a fairly new phenomenon. This involves a major and quite difficult surgical operation to implant electrodes in the lower part of the spinal canal and a radio receiver just beneath the skin over the lower ribs. The bladder is then emptied by holding an appropriate radio transmitter over the implanted receiver.

Victoria, one of two women who have had a bladder implant, replied to the question about how incontinence affected her life. 'It doesn't!! (Yippee), but it did. It almost totally dominated my life, but I have had a bladder controller implant and it has changed everything. It is superb, I never have to think about my bladder, toilet access, plastic pants, pads, etc.'

The prospect of this solution to the problems of incontinence is providing a lot of hope for some of us. Deborah applied to have an implant 'as soon as I heard about it because I will do anything to get rid of this problem'.

Others are more cautious. Marie welcomes the development 'but I'm not sure if it is for me. As I have feeling I wonder if it might prove too painful and then I would lose the little control I have. It is still too new. Perhaps later on I will be more confident about it.' She has decided to stay with her indwelling catheter because of the 'problems of finding suitable loos, etc'. Elspeth requested an implant, but after tests her bladder was found to be unsuitable for the operation.

Urinary diversion

A urinary diversion (urinary or ileal conduit, sometimes called a urostomy) is the solution of last resort but has worked out well for the 11 women who have had one. It involves major surgery. Urine is diverted from the bladder by transplanting the ureters into an isolated loop of small intestine which is then brought out through the wall of the abdomen and urine is collected in a bag. All of us shy away from the thought of such a permanent assault on our bodies. But the misery caused by the failure of other methods of bladder control meant that the women who had had a urinary diversion were pleased they had done so.

Miriam, who became paralysed as the result of arachnoiditis (a progressive disease of the membrane covering the spinal cord), has had an ileal conduit for the last eight years and has found it much easier to cope with as there is 'no more hunting for accessible loos often urgently needed'. She had had an indwelling catheter for four years before that but found 'My urethra became stretched and catheters kept slipping out . . . The surgery for the ileal conduit was traumatic, due to complications – but otherwise, after it was over, I felt it was a wise move.'

Mabel had a urinary diversion in 1984. 'I changed from a catheter after having had lots of trouble being wet, having to use lots of pads. Then infections. So when the stoma [urinary diversion] was discussed I decided that would be better for me and have had absolutely no trouble at all. I was in hospital for one month and took a while to pick up again, but it was worthwhile.'

Pads and pants

The unreliability of the majority of methods of coping with urinary incontinence for women meant that most, though by no means all, of us use some form of incontinence pants and pads to try to prevent our incontinence from becoming too public. One of the most telling indictments of the incontinence industry's products is the finding that almost as many women take the time and trouble to make their own incontinence pads as those who use manufactured ones. Most of these home-made pads are made out of cotton wool surrounding cellulose wadding and covered in gauze, with the supplies obtained on doctor's prescriptions from the chemist. As Lindy declared, 'In all these years I have never found any manufactured pads which did the job better than home-made ones.'

Comments about manufactured pads were not flattering. Paula gave up using pads because they were 'so bulky and not even reliable'. A number of us complained of the size and Hilary made a plea for 'better shaped pads'. Lauren finds pads 'very uncomfortable' and Phyllis would like to see softer inco-rolls because 'some inco pads tear the skin off you'.

Our collective experience of the inadequacies of the pads available indicates an area of enormous need where consumers have become resigned to not being asked what they really want and putting up with what is available.

'The whole family knew when I was wearing them . . . !' Not surprisingly, that was sufficient reason for Willa to stop wearing incontinence pants as 'they crinkle when you move'. Despite the social drawbacks, however, many of us find we have to wear incontinence pants so that we do not get embarrassed by being wet.

The inadequacy of the market in matching people's needs is even more marked in respect of pants than it is for pads. A

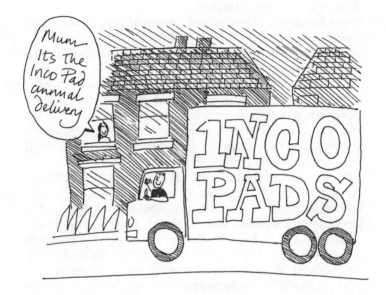

number of us regret that certain makes of pants are no longer being manufactured. Marie echoes the complaints of many of us: 'I would like to see improved plastic that doesn't make you so hot and uncomfortable but does the same job.'

The unsuitability of all the available manufactured incontinence pants has led some of us to make our own, like Christine. 'I make pants by cutting up plastic pants and sewing the bottom half into Marks and Spencer's cotton pants. Thus there is less sweat and heat than using the whole plastic pant, which is unnecesary for me.'

Not only do manufacturers not produce what we want, but there's a further limitation placed on meeting our needs by the narrow range of supplies carried locally – whether by the social services or health services as local providers of incontinence supplies. As Judith says, 'I would like to see a wide range [of goods] carried by social services because what suits one does not suit another.'

What affects bladder incontinence?
The initial shock of having lost control of your bladder, and your bewilderment at its totally random behaviour, becomes ameliorated over time as you gradually learn what is likely to affect the way in which your bladder works. As our replies demonstrated, there is no particular set of rules – and what can affect one person drastically has no effect on another. However, certain patterns related to particular drinks, foods and sets of circumstances emerge from the replies, which are helpful in the context of the continual guessing game of what one's bladder is likely to do next.

'Beer goes straight through me!' Marie's comment speaks for many of us who find that wine and beer tend to have an immediate effect on incontinence. Spirits, however, tend to have the reverse effect and cause dehydration, as Deborah comments: 'Gin – helps incontinence but doesn't do much for the kidneys!' Liz summed it up, saying 'Alcohol upsets my bladder in contradictory ways – sometimes causing retention; other times increasing the flow'. The only solution offered (apart from total abstinence) came from Theresa that 'Eating with drinks absorbs it longer'.

'I find coffee affects my bladder. I found this out a few years ago and have never drunk coffee since' – Janet names the other drink which causes the most problems. Drinking no, or less, coffee can cause some restrictions socially, as Katherine points out: 'Can't drink coffee when I'm out – it goes in one end and straight out the other in a flood! Have to drink tea or not drink at all and then fill up with gallons of water when I get home.'

'I have to avoid late night drinks,' comments Abigail, and that was the case for many of our respondents. Tessa finds: 'I can drink hot chocolate before I go to bed without getting up in the night but nothing else after about 8 p.m.' Theresa put it briefly, 'milk drinks stay in longer.'

The greatest contrasts were in reaction to acidic drinks. Phyllis said: 'I keep off acid drinks and drink plenty of good clean water to help flush my bladder out.' Helen has found 'Drinking regular glasses of lemon and lime diluted squash keeps my urine clear and helps my catheter to last longer.'

Alison wrote of other causes of incontinence: 'I haven't noticed food or drink making a difference – but oncoming colds and tummy upsets have a markedly bad effect. Also, three years ago I had radiotherapy on breast lumps and this had a bad effect on my waterworks. I've had infections on numerous occasions since, which I never had before.'

The effect of the menstrual cycle on incontinence was, however, the factor mentioned by most of us, the majority finding menstruation made incontinence more likely. For most of us it is the days just before menstruation which tend to be the most uncontrollable. Magda finds: 'I usually have "accidents" just before my period starts.' Hilary linked this to the fact that she is more constipated at this time. For some, the days before our period tend to be easier than normal because we are more inclined to retention. But this stores up trouble for a few days later on. Theresa finds: 'My menstrual cycle causes havoc. Usually about three to four days before it I pass less water, then more during my period, and at erratic times.'

Bridget went to a homoeopath in desperation when she found that constantly needing to pee during the first 48 hours of her period was making her working life impossible. In spite of her scepticism the homoeopathic remedy she was given has so far completely solved this problem.

Bowels

Very few of us find that bowel incontinence is as much of a problem as bladder incontinence. The lack of feeling and/or control over this bodily function means that we have to rely on a mixture of routine, diet and stimulation (suppositories and/or manual evacuation). There are, however, a number of problems associated with bowel incontinence.

We are all different and need to sort out what is best for our bodies and individual life styles, rather than fit into the particular regime of the spinal unit we initially attended. Our own feelings about bowel incontinence may also be a problem, although very few of us actually expressed the distress felt by Dawn who finds doing a manual evacuation 'awful and degrading'. Another major problem for some was the time that it takes to move the bowels, sometimes up to one-and-a-half to two hours. And, of course, 'accidents' are unpredictable. This fear can loom large. Julia wrote: 'If there is an accident, I do tend to fall apart and feel very embarrassed . . . It has not happened to me away from home – it is something I try not to think about.'

Sorting things out for ourselves

Liz found, like many of us, that the spinal unit imposed an 'every other day' routine, which she abandoned immediately she left. 'I radically changed my diet to one that is vegetarian/wholefood/high fibre. My routine is daily. Experience has shown that the bowel empties in "waves", with pauses in between. After the first "wave" I use more suppositories and repeat the process until I'm happy the bowel has nothing more to dispose of. I use a finger sometimes to relax the anal muscles and to check the rectum is clear before getting off the loo. Above all, I take my time – about an hour! – while I can wash, partially dress and do my hair. Wine, cider and beer are all to be avoided in any quantity as I've found they set the bowels in rapid motion.' Her advice is: 'By observing an exacting morning routine you can liberate yourself from the fear of soiling yourself when socialising, or asleep in bed, or indeed at any time.'

Bridget, on the other hand, does not have any particular routine or take a very long time. 'Each time I go for a pee, I insert a finger into my vagina which tells me if my lower bowel needs emptying. If it does I use my finger. I find it takes less time than it used to before I was paralysed! I have only once had an accident – when I had diarrhoea.'

Tessa also has few problems with this aspect of paralysis. 'If I eat Weetabix, three slices of wholemeal bread and a banana per day (or equivalent) I rarely need suppositories or laxatives. After breakfast my bowels will either open within a few minutes or it'll almost certainly be the following day.

By putting a little pressure just in front of the anus, the stool just slides out. The only time I can expect problems is just before my menstrual cycle when I always get constipated.'

Most of us are told we should move our bowels in the morning. Mary, however, finds that she does not have time in the morning 'so I go at night and it works just as well'. Martha also goes in the evening: 'every other evening between 9 p.m. and 12 p.m. It takes 30 minutes to one hour. If nothing happens, at least I have all night to see if anything is going to, so I sleep on an inco pad. So far – touch wood – no accident during the day.'

Valerie, paralysed in 1955, manages without help, even though her hands are paralysed. 'I insert Dulcolax suppositories with a suppository inserter every other morning 20 minutes before transferring to a toilet, and sit for an hour tapping the left side of my abdomen when I get a head flush sensation and my bowel clears itself without manual evacuation. The only laxative I use is Fibogel. I hardly ever have an accident these days. I eat plenty of fibre in my diet.'

The majority of us have found that we get to know what pattern and diet suits our body best, and many are able to echo Linda when she says 'I cope extremely well', although she could only say this once she left the spinal unit.

Pauline was the only one of us to have had a colostomy. She initially had one because of the internal injuries which she experienced as a result of the car accident which left her an incomplete tetraplegic. The colostomy could have been reversed, but she chose not to have this done. 'I can cope well with it and it is now a personal thing. I can change it [the bag] myself. I don't have to stick to any particular diet. I would certainly recommend it.'

Depending on others

Bowel incontinence is, however, one aspect of paralysis which for some of us (particularly for tetraplegics) can mean dependence on others. Usually the district or community nurse will come in to do a manual evacuation, although

Esme feels that 'this is an aspect the community nurse would rather not deal with as if it is not part of paraplegia'. Dependence on an outsider means that you have to wait for them to come, and a frequent complaint is the irregularity of their visits and that they cannot fit you in to their routines to suit you.

Our feelings about this reliance on others vary. Chloe thinks that she and her Mum 'cope very well'. But Geraldine, paralysed at the age of 13 at the level of C5/6, found it very difficult being dependent on her mother. 'I hated this,' she wrote, 'because I was a very independent person and it made me feel like a baby.'

Do we have time for anything else . . . ?
Those of us who find that moving our bowels can take a long time have to find ways of fitting the rest of our lives around this. Alison gets up at 6.40 a.m. every morning, while Liz makes sure that she allows at least an hour in the morning.

Christine finds that bowel incontinence threatens her ability to pursue her working life. 'In the last few years – about since I was 40 and I am now 48 – I have had bowel troubles which, if I had still been in the classroom, would probably have forced me to give up work. Being a college lecturer by this time, I manage to organise my days and life so as to minimise disruption in this way. It is still a problem but has not (yet) proved insuperable.'

Cora finds that she has to: 'set aside two nights a week to deal with this and never spend a night away from home unless bowels have been emptied first. I feel that I cannot safely leave home for more than a week.' For her and for some others, bowel incontinence means limitations and restrictions. Amanda, for example, describes the restrictions on her life. At home her bowel incontinence is under control by using Dulcolax liquid every other night with the help of a nurse or her mother, but this makes going away with friends impossible – 'So I don't go away'.

Conclusion

The most important message seems to be that incontinence, and particularly bladder incontinence, is one of the most significant impacts of spinal cord injury. Yet it is too often a problem which is hidden away, and it has been found to be very difficult to work together with the medical and ancillary professions to sort out individual solutions to individual problems.

Having said this, a number of us (usually without the professional help we need) have managed to sort out systems for dealing with incontinence which prevent this dominating our lives. Moreover, we often find that the realities of incontinence become less humiliating over the years, and that those who are close to us also cease to find it embarrassing. What may seem to be insurmountable problems when we are newly paralysed, become, with experience, possible to deal with. Unfortunately, we are too often thrown back on our own wits and resources in confronting this major aspect of our lives, as usually medical and social services professionals have little help to offer.

11.

Medical Complications

Among the 205 women who returned the questionnaire are found the same range of health problems that one would expect to find in a sample of a similar number of non-disabled people. However, in addition to these, we experience a number of medical complications which may be a direct result of paralysis. The intention is not to provide a textbook discussion of these medical complications but rather to share our experience of them. It must be stressed, however, that if the reader is looking for accurate medical information, she should consult either one of the books in the bibliography or contact a spinal unit (addresses and telephone numbers are in the Resources list). The Spinal Injuries Association can also help in gaining access to information (see the address and telephone number in the Resources list).

As newly disabled women we often contemplate the future with fears of ill health and increasing dependency. It is, of course, difficult to know just how representative of spinal cord injured women our group of 205 women are but, for the most part, our experiences do not bear out these fears. Moira, for example was paralysed in 1953 and, apart from a few pressure sores in her early years of disability, did not return to hospital for 28 years. There are a number of health problems which are specifically related to our paralysis but for very few of us have these constituted a major threat to our ways of living. It is notable, in fact, how little most of us have had to say in answer to the question on medical complications. However, amongst those of us who did have problems in this area, six distinct types of difficulty could be distinguished.

Bladders and kidneys

Urinary tract infections (UTIs) are a common problem associated with incontinence and were mentioned by one in four of us. Difficulties in emptying the bladder properly can cause infections, and some doctors believe the use of catheters (indwelling or intermittent) can also lead to bladder infections. Kidney infections can result from bladder infections if we have reflux – that is, when the valves which stop urine backflowing from the ureters to the kidneys weaken and the infection therefore spreads to the kidneys. Most of us who experience UTIs rely on antibiotics, but some have successfully prevented their recurrence by taking measures such as those recommended in Angela Kilmartin's book *Understanding Cystitis*; particularly emptying the bladder completely, avoiding coffee and spirits, and being careful about personal hygiene.

An associated problem is bladder or kidney stones, and these were mentioned by 14 women. They result from a build-up of calcium in the bladder or kidney and can be removed either surgically or through laser treatment.

Pressure and other skin problems

A fear of pressure sores is usually drummed into us while we are in the spinal unit, and they are certainly one of the commonest health hazards associated with paralysis. One in four of us mentioned having pressure sores. A sore is usually caused by pressure (from sitting or lying) being exerted for too long on one point, thus reducing blood supply and damaging underlying tissue. Further complications can set in if an abscess develops which can then infect the bone. (This was experienced by eight women.) Once this has happened we need immediate admission to a spinal unit where treatment may involve removal of the infected piece of bone and plastic surgery. This will certainly involve many weeks, sometimes months, of keeping off the pressure point. We are constantly told that the only way to prevent pressure sores is to keep a beady eye open for any red marks on the bottom, heel, foot, etc. and to keep pressure completely off such marks when they occur. Many of us, however, find days or weeks of keeping off our bottoms impossible (how can we carry on working and/or looking after our family, etc?) and have developed our own ways of dealing with such problems – sometimes successfully and sometimes not. These include using a Roho cushion (an air-filled cushion) or cutting holes at the appropriate point in a foam cushion.

An associated problem is bursars, which are cushions of fluid which tend to develop over bony prominences; these are also experienced by non-disabled people. They cause problems if the pressure is not released and more fluid is produced which can then turn septic. As with pressure sores, the long-term, and preventive, solution is to reduce the pressure on vulnerable areas. Hazel is one of the very few of us who has experienced serious problems with bursars. 'In 14 years I can count on two hands the times I've been in [hospital] with bursars,' she says. Happily, a Roho cushion seems to have solved the problem.

Our loss of sensation can also mean that we unwittingly burn ourselves on a radiator, sitting too close to a fire, etc. Eight of us mentioned having problems with burns – they can, of course, take a long time to heal and cause major inconvenience.

Circulatory conditions

Our reduced mobility means that we may experience complications associated with a sluggish blood flow. These include thrombosis in the calf of the leg (experienced by 10 of us). Another problem, oedema, the swelling of feet and ankles and in some women the lower part of the legs, is mainly a problem of appearance rather than a serious threat to health. Chilblains can also result from poor circulation and can be guarded against by keeping warm. More seriously, poor circulation can also mean that cuts and bruises take longer to heal, and may be more likely to become infected. Finally, hypothermia is a risk, particularly for tetraplegic women who get less warning if their body temperature is getting dangerously low. However, only one of us had experienced hypothermia.

Respiratory problems

If our level of injury means that our chest and lungs are affected we may find it difficult or impossible to cough, and this can have quite serious implications in the event of a cold. Five women mentioned such problems. Chest infections can quickly turn into bronchitis and pneumonia if not treated with antibiotics and/or physiotherapy. Vicky, a tetraplegic, wrote about two bouts of pneumonia: 'both were worse than they needed to be because the GP didn't appreciate the implications of a chest infection until nearly too late.'

Contractures, arthritis and scoliosis

Our bodies were not designed to sit in a wheelchair or use crutches, and not surprisingly long-term use of either can lead to problems such as contractures (where the tendons shorten and prevent the proper movement of the legs, feet or arms). Osteoarthritis can result from the overuse of the joints on which we rely to maintain mobility and nine of us mentioned that we had developed some form of arthritis although at least some of us would have developed such a condition even if not disabled. Sarah writes that she now has 'osteoarthritis on nearly all weight-bearing joints, plus complications'. She advises: 'don't overstrain the limbs you are still able to use unless you have an ambition to be an

Olympic champion; measure active life and the muscles you have to use.'

Poor posture while sitting in a wheelchair can lead to scoliosis where the spine becomes crooked. Cynthia, paraplegic since 1959, has found that, 'Due to my sitting position I am now badly twisted and attending a clinic to try to improve my posture. I would like to warn new lesions of the importance of sitting well.' Geraldine, an incomplete tetraplegic, found that her scoliosis required surgery, a rod being put in to straighten her spine.

Fourteen of us had had broken bones, usually a leg. This can result from a combination of weaker bones and the increased vulnerability arising from the lack of sensation and the possibility of falling awkwardly while on crutches or using a wheelchair.

Spasms

Most of us have spasms [involuntary muscle contractions] in our paralysed limbs of some kind; these sometimes serve a purpose such as warning us when our bladders need emptying or preventing muscle wastage. For 29 of us spasms have caused big problems. Madeline, for example, found that the nature of her spasms changed over the years. Injured in 1964 at C7/T3, she writes, 'I had a complete change of spasms from helpful enjoyable extensor spasms to incessant flexor spasms – dangerous because I couldn't brake when driving, exhausting because they went on, day and night, nasty because I saw myself becoming less independent (could hardly get out of the bath, etc.). I had an alcohol block [an operation on the spinal cord] which was a success (I still spasm and have become more spastic again over the years, but they're not overwhelming).'

Meeting our needs

One of the major problems associated with health problems

for us is whether GPs and general hospitals know enough about spinal cord injury and its effects to give us appropriate treatment. Furthermore, both the physical environment within a hospital and its nursing practices can deprive us of independence. The lack of a wheelchair-accessible lavatory on a hospital ward has major implications. It is not unknown for wheelchairs to be removed once someone is admitted to a general hospital, thus denying that person any independence.

We are at the same risk as the rest of the population of having non-paralysis-related health probems, and any admission to hospital, for example, for breast cancer, can be made a particularly difficult experience if there are inadequate facilities and ignorance of the needs of paraplegics and tetraplegics. Our best experiences of general hospitals are when their staff recognise we are experts in our everyday personal care and allow and/or enable us to continue whatever daily routines we have. Jackie writes: 'I would like to see doctors and nurses realise the fact that when you are paralysed for a long period you know your body better than they do ... the disabled person is in many instances more aware of her body's needs than the people who are treating her.'

Karen found that this aspect of hospitalisation was indeed appreciated by her general hospital: 'I was well looked after and my guidelines for prevention of bedsores were understood. The nurses appreciated that I was independent and knew I understood how to care for myself. I got lots of support and kindness.' All too often, however, we have had to be 'rescued' by spinal units from inappropriate treatment in general hospitals, which sometimes, for example, results in pressure sores which take many months to heal.

Some of the worst experiences result from medical practitioners' failure to recognise that we cannot rely on pain as a warning signal. Thus, Beth found that her broken leg went untreated for two years 'because I couldn't feel it and the GP refused to X-ray it because if it didn't hurt [he said] it couldn't be broken ... ' Injured in 1955, Beth seems to have had more health problems than most of us – 'I've broken each leg, been in and out of hospital with pressure sores, foot infections, burns due to not noticing I was exposed to heat, etc.' However, she goes on to say, 'My initial dread of spending my life in and out of hospital with relapses has been unfounded.'

For those whose disability has brought health problems, the experience is often one of becoming disillusioned with professional care and gradually taking more and more responsibility for their own bodies. This is true for Margery, an incomplete paraplegic since 1961, who writes, 'In the 1960s and 1970s I was in and out of hospital like a yoyo. Mainly through trying to do too much physically. In 1977 I was finally given a firm list of don'ts and accepted that physical effort was not for me. I have sought relief from pain through many orthodox and unorthodox sources – unsuccessfully. Have had many minor but long-lasting pressure sores and spend at least part of each year on antibiotics. Have now been told to stay on low dosage permanently. Doctors – and nurses – are always in a hurry, have no time to listen and care nothing for the prevention of illness unless it can be solved by taking a pill. I now make an effort to stay away from doctors and hospitals and am becoming more and more interested in alternative or fringe medicine.'

The overall picture obtained from the section of the questionnaire dealing with medical complications is that we are often driven to find possible solutions ourselves to the health problems we have – a positive step in many ways but, even so, we could do with more constructive help from the professionals concerned.

12.

Pain

Pain, a small word with many implications. For some of us pain permeates all aspects of our lives: our family, work, social and sexual lives. It is an intrusive by-product of spinal injury which has the potential to damage us physically, emotionally and socially. At worst, our daily lives are reduced to an existence centred around pain. Otherwise, it may stretch both patience and wits, as we seek ways to keep the intrusions of pain at bay. Only a minority of us are free to 'enjoy' disability without it.

Pain has no respect for levels of lesion; whether the lesions are complete or incomplete; what age we were when we were injured; whether the injury was caused by trauma, tumour or virus. Our wonderful bodies – with that incredibly complicated central nervous system which is the locus of our shared experience – react with a vengeance when they are damaged. Yet maybe just knowing that we are not alone helps us to gain strength. Maybe the sharing of our experience of pain, and learning from and growing in understanding through each other, will also help. Maybe this will in fact give us the strength to start to demand positive action on pain: for example, more research into its causes, relief and management.

What are we talking about?

Where is the pain? The short answer, judging from our responses, is anywhere or everywhere. The degrees of aching,

burning or discomfort that come within our physical descriptions of pain seem to be experienced in just about every
part of our bodies. One in four of us experience pain which
is so serious that it curtails our activities or confines us to
bed for all or part of the time. Pain does not seem to follow
any set pattern for any particular level of lesion, whether
cervical, thoracic or lumbar, or whether complete or incomplete.

Certain types of pain can, however, be distinguished.

Root pain

Root pain is pain that comes from the parts of our bodies
which no longer experience normal sensation. Daisy, who
tersely describes her 'very severe root pain for 10 years', is
talking about a jangled message passed through to the brain
by damaged nerves. As such, it is incredibly difficult to describe or, for those who do not experience it, to understand.
Nadia describes her root pain as 'a burning sensation up and
down my legs which occurs 24 hours a day'. Christine says:
'My behind gets sore (which is weird since I can't feel it)
when I sit too much so I try to lie down when I can which is
not terribly often!' She is relatively lucky in that the pain will
respond to some action, as will Nadia's root pain which she
treats with distalgesics at bedtime because otherwise she
cannot sleep. Irene, however, says that the root pain in her
right foot has blighted her life and 'no pills touch root pain
which increases with age'.

Brenda describes how root pain, together with cramps
and backache, has been the 'real complication' following
her incomplete tetraplegia. 'It started in hospital, about a
month after the accident, in the feet, working up the legs to
waist height – at that time a feeling of intense cold. Since
then the sensations have changed to acute stomach cramps,
backache and burning legs. At times the combination of all
three becomes very hard to bear. Otherwise there is always
a feeling of general discomfort and now I am always very
conscious of my feet. Until about six months ago all I wanted

was to sleep as I didn't feel it then. The GP tried me on various drugs and then referred me to a pain clinic. More drugs without conspicuous success and the end of what could be tried. The biggest help was being taught by my GP how to forcibly relax, a form of self-hypnosis. Now a mixture of lying flat on the floor, forcibly relaxing or keeping myself as occupied as possible (even only reading the paper helps). Again, [during] the last three or four months it has changed in kind and is generally more liveable with.'

Anita also has a lot to say about root pain. A tetraplegic, injured 17 years ago, she writes, 'Yes, I have suffered pain. The doctors call it root pain. It is hard to describe because it is so diverse. It is very difficult to describe the excruciating pain to many people. The common reaction from professionals and lay people is: "If you can't feel, how can you have pain?" This is very upsetting. Most professionals know about the phantom pain that amputees suffer, so why can they not accept that we have a great deal of pain, even though there may be no sensory feeling? The pain started as soon as I was paralysed, got worse and has stayed constantly with me for the last 17 years. I don't cope very well. Some days it is worse than others. No matter what I am doing I am always aware of it. Sometimes it gets so bad I cannot cope and have to go away into a corner and cry. No painkillers touch it. Smoking sometimes helps – it sort of numbs it. Alcohol numbs it as well, but if alcohol has a depressant effect on the brain cells that may be the reason that it helps the pain. I feel that the pain does affect my life; it makes me feel very depressed at times and when it is severe I don't go out because the bumping in the wheelchair makes it worse. The pain is from my waist downwards and doesn't miss any area out.'

Rosalind is someone else whose life is made difficult by root pain. 'I get very bad root pain which gets worse when I am tired, ill or under stress. It affects the whole of my lower half and often feels as though someone is giving me electric shocks. It started in hospital but got much worse. I tried acupuncture, electrodes etc. I find it very difficult to cope with . . . One of the greatest problems is trying to explain what it is like to other people. Because it is not like ordinary pain it's very difficult to describe. I find only other paraplegics who get it can really understand – and even then the degree of severity varies a lot.'

Hypersensitivity

Hypersensitivity is another type of pain which will only sometimes respond to painkillers. Wendy has hypersensitivity in her legs, arms and fingers. She says 'I took tablets at first but gave them up when I found out they were not having much effect. Some days the hypersensitivity can be worse than others with all my body tingling.' Marie (with an incomplete T5 lesion) has a hypersensitive hand and 'cannot bear the sheets touching it at night or wearing any rings on the fingers'.

Sometimes hypersensitivity disappears after the first few weeks or months of paralysis. Bridget, for example, found that the hypersensitivity on her abdomen lasted no more than a few weeks. 'I do however have a patch of skin on my back which unpredictably, but at infrequent intervals, becomes very very sore.' Medical explanation of this type of hypersensitivity tends to be that 'it is the damaged nerves protesting' and few of us have received much help with the problem.

Aches and pains

There is the pain which is associated with difficulties with our backs and necks, or general muscular problems. Sometimes there is an identifiable reason, as with Marie who had a metal plate put in her back following her injury. 'I've always had the pain in my back from the steel plate,' she says, 'but it gets worse when I'm tired or ill. I ignore it because drugs don't affect the pain.'

Those of us who walk with crutches and/or calipers often find that their use can cause pain. Margery, an incomplete L1 lesion, found that using crutches caused pain and numbness in her arms and hands and pain in neck and shoulders. Libby, walking with a stick following a dislocation of her C4 and C5 vertebrae, has 'a fair amount of back and neck pain (due to stiffness and spasticity) and pain of the joints generally, hips in particular. I have found that going to a physiotherapist who practises "Touch for Health" and does massages and osteopathy (as well as using herbal remedies and advising on diet) has been very helpful.'

Leila experienced pain in her knee for some time, and her general hospital 'told me there was nothing they could do – I'd just have to live with it.' She referred herself to a spinal unit where they immediately recognised that, although she was walking, she had developed a contracture of the tendon behind her knee. The solution was simply to stretch the tendon and the pain which had got 'so bad, I didn't want to fight any more' disappeared. Similarly, Pamela, who can also walk, finds that the spasms in her trunk muscles can cause them to tighten up. The pain resulting from this is soon dealt with by a week or so of physiotherapy.

Often, though, it is not clear what the cause is. Phyllis writes: 'My pain is chiefly in my spine, arms and shoulders. Sometimes I think I will go crackers, but usually after a couple of days in bed, keeping very warm – well the top half of me anyhow, I manage to push the pain out of my mind. I think I have a very high pain threshold now.'

Damage to muscles and joints through overuse and arthritis are mentioned by some of us who have been paralysed for some years. Margery, injured in 1961, writes, 'I already have arthritis in damaged areas which will probably get worse with age.' Valerie finds that, after 30 years of being a tetraplegic, she is now starting to get pain in her shoulders and neck. She finds that lying on her stomach at night helps, as do sitting straight in the chair and daily exercise of neck and shoulder muscles.

Some of us experience trapped nerves, including sciatica, and other back problems. Sarah, paralysed in 1958 at the level of T10/11, has 'severe pain in my lower back from pressure on certain nerves due to collapsed discs, including pressure on sciatic nerve with general pain when sitting as a result of my degenerating joints. The problems began in 1977 and have gradually been getting worse. I take painkillers which only work partially. At times I can only cope by lying on the bed for an hour or two, to take the pressure off the spine and pelvis. I now have to measure out my activity for each day in order to remain as productive as possible.'

Beryl writes: 'My problem is the terrible (referred) nerve pain in my lower spine, which is caused by trapped nerves in scar tissue in my higher back.' Mavis had a tumour removed from her spine in 1963 and has become progressively paralysed. She has pain from a trapped nerve in her back which she controls with diazepan. 'When I cannot cope,' she says, 'I take an occasional palfium. I don't like resorting to palfium as I feel I am giving in to the pain, but my consultants, my doctor and others say that I am wearing myself out and must allow myself a break from the severity which is sometimes very bad.'

Spasms and pain

Spasms are involuntary muscle contractions in the paralysed parts of the body, and a number of us find that they are the cause of pain. Olivia writes: 'I used to get terribly strong spasm in my legs, which threw me forward in my chair and nearly out of it on some occasions. It used to hurt my stomach. I used to take Dantrium tablets but decided to give these up as the spasm seemed to be growing weaker of its own accord.'

Liz wrote that she does not have pain as such but experiences 'grinding, wearing exhaustion which comes from periods of *acute* discomfort when every part of you aches and something is spasming more violently than usual, preventing true rest or sleep. This seems to sap my strength in a very demoralising manner.' For Pauline, spasms have both advantages and disadvantages. She writes: 'I get painful spasms, but accept them as part of my disability – I take Baclofen to control them. Without these spasms I would have an awful lot of muscle wastage so, in their own way, they are quite a blessing.'

How does pain affect our lives?

Rosalind writes about her root pain, 'It affects my life a lot. I often have to decline invitations, either because I'm in too much pain, or because I may already be tired and can't risk getting more tired (and more pain). This is depressing. At work it often affects my concentration and I have had to lie down or leave early. I avoid long car journeys because they make me more tired . . . I do try not to let it rule my life and I do get some relatively good days when I don't really notice it much.'

Erica writes about how pain has affected her daily life. 'Pain has been the biggest factor throughout the time I have been disabled. Travel irritates the pain so I try to limit time in a car, etc. Any long journeys which are unavoidable, my GP prescribes Pethedine to help. From listening to family and friends' comments, if the pain is very bad I become withdrawn and almost put shutters round myself which sometimes leaves them feeling useless.' She continues, 'Because the pain prevents me from sleeping, my husband and I have agreed to sleep in separate rooms, as if I lie awake he becomes upset and then he too has a sleepless night. Both of us hate this arrangement but agree it is the most sensible. Pain affects my attitude towards love-making. Pain puts up its own limitations and there are many occasions when I am unable to do what I planned or go where I'd planned. As the level fluctuates, it is difficult to make long-term plans or any real commitment to any project which inevitably leads to frustrations and resentment.'

Erica's final comment sums it all up: 'I've always maintained that if they could control the pain there would be no problem as the wheelchair is no big deal.'

What can we do about it?

Many of us complained about the response of the medical profession or physiotherapists to our experience of pain. Often we are told to just 'put up with it'. It seems particularly difficult to get professionals to take root pain seriously; Gillian gave up trying to get help with her root problem. 'I've learnt to try and cope with it,' she wrote, 'as the medics don't believe it's there.'

Nadine, injured in 1981 at the level of T3/4, wrote about her fears and the lack of help. 'I get loss of sensation and pain in my fingers and arms mainly in bed at night. It has happened occasionally ever since the accident, but got worse after about two years. The spinal unit has not given any explanation or treatment. I have not been able to discover what causes it. Sometimes it happens frequently, sometimes it does not happen for several weeks. Although the pain can be very intense, it usually lasts only a few minutes. If it causes lack of sleep it can make me tired and irritable and I sometimes worry about it and get depressed.'

Root pain is sometimes affected by drugs or may be eased by other treatment such as that which Geraldine describes. 'I get a lot of root pain in my right leg. I find if someone rubs the back of my neck it eventually goes.' Martha finds that her solution to pain can be embarrassing. 'The only pain I have,' she writes, 'is in my right breast. It's a sharp but fluctuating pain that I've had ever since the accident. It doesn't really affect me except that to release it I have to press it – which doesn't look too good in company!'

As Erica has described, pain is the dominating factor in her life and she has a constant battle in dealing with it. 'It is like toothache,' she writes, 'and I find it very tiring. I can't really say when this severe pain began exactly, but it developed after surgery and myelograms [X-rays of the spinal cord after fluid has been injected into the spinal column]. Sometimes it is severe enough to make me vomit and I have fainted on two occasions. I try to cope but people, including some doctors, can't understand that the pain never changes but my "copability" does. I'm a great believer in filling my mind and days as much as possible in an effort to push the pain to the back of my mind. It doesn't always work but is much better than giving in. If it's dreadful, I remind myself that pain can't kill – although there have been times that I have wished it did! I spend most afternoons doing something I can lie almost flat doing as I find sitting very painful. I administer injections of Tangesic as and when I need them and the amount varies according to what I am doing. Usually it's about 1 ml × 3mg. every four to six hours. I don't take it at night so my body has a break from the drug. I also take drugs to help me sleep, but even on a high dose I only manage two to three hours each night – i.e. the drugs help me to go off to sleep but the pain wakes me. I still take the drugs as on waking although the pain is bad I am more relaxed following sleep so more able to cope without the use of analgesia.'

Rosalind also has to limit her activities according to the amount of pain she is experiencing. She finds that: 'Sometimes the only way to push it into the background is to try and get involved in something active: cooking, cleaning, etc. . . . I have tried some pain-killing drugs but am very reluctant to take many. I do find that whisky (and soda) helps take the edge off the root pain!'

Sometimes physiotherapy can help if the pain is owing to poor posture. Unfortunately, Lindy found that she had to pay for private physiotherapy in her own home as going to the local hospital for treatment was too traumatic, particularly as the hospital staff will not allow her to use her own wheelchair in the hospital. Beth was told that her very bad backache was untreatable and would be constant. However, she found that 'daily swimming, yoga and Alexander technique have cured it'.

Some of us are lucky enough to find that if we keep our minds on something else other than root pain it does not bother us too much. Bridget (a college lecturer) says, 'The only time I don't notice the burning sensation I have in my legs and bottom is when I'm lecturing. At other times, it's just there at the back of my perception as long as I don't actually focus on it. Immediately I think about it, like now writing about it, it becomes all pervading.'

Amelia, who broke her back at L1/2 in 1951, has been relatively successful in dealing with her pain, although initially everything failed to make an impact. She tried hydrotherapy, acupuncture, nerve blocks and, as a last resort, hypnotism. 'At first,' she says, 'I didn't cope very well but then I realised that they weren't going to be able to do anything to relieve the pain and it was either going to rule my life or I had to get on top of it. I can't do as much as I used to and there are times when I have to give in and lie down and keep very still.'

Sometimes, surgical intervention can solve the problem of pain, as Vicky found. She says she was 'heading straight for a nervous breakdown when the situation changed after major surgery to my spinal cord. The operations were about 85 per cent successful and now I can cope with the pain that is left.' Esme, though, has not been so lucky in her search for a solution. 'I've had investigations by neurologists but so far they cannot account for it. I've tried the "black box" pain-killer [an electronic treatment] and various tablets which haven't had any long-term effects. Pain in my back and shoulders lately is bad after sitting for longer periods than I'm used to. I am due to see a neurologist again soon. I've had X-rays on my hips two years ago, but nothing was diagnosed which could be dealt with by surgery.' Lillian discovered that her district health authority runs a pain clinic, but so far they have not found a solution for her problem, as she writes, 'Constant pain wears one out.'

Others have found that changing to a new wheelchair can make a big difference, although some find that the only solution is to lie down. Margery never sits if she can lie down, and even travels in a reclining seat with pillows. 'I can now stand a level of pain which would have had me laid out moaning 10 years ago,' she writes.

Not all spinal cord injured women experience pain, but it does seem to be fairly common. One in four of those answering the questionnaire (51 women) experience serious pain (that is, the pain prevents us from taking part in things or confines us to bed for all or part of the time). Another 76 women gave details of how pain affected their lives. Our most common experience of reactions to our pain is, unfortunately, that there is not much that anyone else can do for us. The medical profession either does not take the problem seriously, or, even if it does, cannot help most of us. What solutions there are to the problem of pain we have usually found for ourselves. We use drugs, physiotherapy and relaxation. We have to adjust our lives around pain, to learn what makes it worse, to continually battle against it taking over our lives.

Many have found there is little we can do to alleviate the pain. Samantha says of the severe pain she gets in her neck and shoulders, 'I just learnt to live with it.'

Conclusion

This is the first book of its kind in this country. It is a book written by spinal cord injured women who want to share their experiences with newly injured women and their friends and relatives, and to impress our concerns upon the general public and professionals. It is part of a growing movement to bring disability issues which previously have been kept private – behind the closed doors of individual lives – out into the open. We hope there will be many more books like this one to follow.

It is no accident that we first approached a feminist publisher. Although many of the women featured in this book would never call themselves feminists, our common concern is to be heard: as women and as disabled women. The Women's Press gives a voice to women who have been silenced, and we are one of the most silenced groups in a society which continues to discriminate in every way against those who do not conform, and do not fit in with the ideal of ability.

For it is an ideal. The physical, economic and social world is organised for a minority; the minority of people who never experience physical difficulties. Most people, at some time in their lives, find out that once their physical capacities, and hence their earning capacities, are diminished, whether through illness, accident, old age or pregnancy, they are at the mercy of a society which does not take such needs into account.

In the Britain of the late 1980s, where community and collective values have been heavily attacked, where the dominant philosophy is very much the survival of the fittest, we are particularly vulnerable. We find the competitive individualism dominant in some spinal units often leaves no room for women; that in order to get suitable housing we rely on collective provision from council or housing association or in the form of improved grants; that we desperately need an efficient and properly resourced health service (including the community health service); that we rely on services and benefits which enable us to get the personal care we need.

A society which is organised so that if you can't pay for it you can't have it, is one in which disabled people find their lives unnecessarily restricted. Disability hits one's earning capacity, and that of one's family, and at the same time means that life is much, much more expensive. The quality of our lives can only worsen when there is inadequate (or no) collective provision – whether in the form of housing, personal services, health care, transport or benefits.

Disability for women raises the particular issues which have been discussed at length in this book. Time and again the material from our questionnaire has demonstrated that medical and social services professionals are not sufficiently aware of these issues. For example, women are primarily the carers within a family and most of us continue in this role. Yet too often it is assumed that we will be the passive recipients of care.

Related to this concern is a failure to recognise that high level tetraplegics can return to independent living – and for many women this means looking after their family – as long as they have someone to be their 'arms and legs'. A physical inability to care for a child does not necessarily mean that we cannot take responsibility for childcare.

Moreover, medical and social services professionals and the general public usually fail to recognise just how much physical ability we have. There are many paraplegic women who look after their children with very little difficulty, and tetraplegic women do as well – there is nothing wrong with lifting a child up by hooking a thumb through a belt (however much it may horrify the health visitor).

Women also often find there are negative reactions to the possibility of their return to independent living if they do not have husbands or parents to care for them. It is standard practice for the health and social services professionals to look to families to care for paraplegics and tetraplegics. This is partly because of the lack of resources available. If a high level tetraplegic is to live independently, she will need a level of personal care which may well not be available other than through the unpaid work of a partner or family. If such unpaid carers are not to hand, women are more likely to end up in residential care, a damning indictment of the philosophy of 'community care'.

All of us, whatever the level of injury, needed a 'package' of alterations to our lives after paralysis. The most common need is suitable housing, but together with the physical characteristics of a house often goes the practical help which makes it possible to live there. This might be in terms of obtaining the state benefits to which we are entitled, getting help with the housework or getting someone to be our arms and legs almost 24 hours a day. Our working lives will also be affected by our disability and we need facilitating action to enable us to continue to earn a living.

A very clear message, which came through the answers to the questionnaire relating to our experience of returning to our lives before injury, was that what advice and support there was available was inadequate, fragmented and unimaginative. It is not surprising that the most helpful support and advice came from other disabled people, because in fact we are the 'experts' on how to rebuild our lives. If only the professionals could learn from our experiences, how much better at their jobs they would be.

The problem is partly a shortage of resources. More fundamentally, it is a problem of attitudes towards disabled people. The dominant reactions to disability are, on the one hand, to ignore the daily and detailed difficulties which we have, and on the other, to make heroes and heroines of those people who achieve some success in struggling against these difficulties. In these days of celebration of the philosophy of 'every man for himself' such attitudes are extremely convenient.

Disabled people are perceived as being either 'wonderful' and 'marvellous' – or inadequate and unable to cope. The rest of society can abdicate responsibility for collective provision as there is a mostly, but not entirely, unspoken belief that some people just can't be helped because they are not 'survivors'. Such an attitude was voiced by the director of a spinal unit, who told Bridget that: 'people either cope with spinal cord injury or they don't – for those who don't have the capacity to cope no amount of support, psychological or material, will make that much difference.'

It is this philosophy – nonsensical though it is – which makes the fight for the resources to enable us to rebuild our lives, so hard. Disability itself does not determine the quality of our lives. Rather, it is the resources available to us which make all the difference. If we have, or can get, the housing and personal care we need, if we have friends and family who value us, occupations (within and outside the home) that we enjoy, then there will be joy in our lives.

We hope that the experiences shared in this book will go some way towards changing the attitudes of the general public and professionals alike. All of us, whether or not we are disabled, need a society which both cares for and values people, whatever their abilities.

Biographies

Set out below is brief information about each of the women whose returned questionnaires we have used to compile this book. Although the statistical analysis of the questionnaires included all 205 returned, we have only quoted from those whose brief biographies are given below. All the names are fictitious. We have tried to give the level of injury, date and age when injured and very brief details about working and family lives. Sometimes this has not been possible, however, because the information provided was incomplete.

The information about level of injury is primarily given because of its interest to women who have been recently injured. It is at this time, when we find out about spinal cord injury and its implications, that 'what level' we are is so important to us. In these early days, we desperately search for information about what other women with the same level of injury are able to do.

We would like to advise the reader not to assume that all these women are white, middle class and heterosexual. Questionnaires were returned by women in a wide variety of occupations and circumstances. They were also returned by women who are black or from an ethnic minority and by women who are lesbians. However, as not all these women identified themselves as such we have not included these details in the biographies.

Abigail: Fell from a window in 1975 when she was 55 years old. T6 incomplete. Walks with sticks. Married and in full-time employment. Now retired.

Adela: Operation in 1979 after years of back problems resulted in paraplegia. 67 years old. Widow. Now in residential care.

Alice: Fall when 24 years old in 1974 resulted in L1/L2 fracture. Walks with sticks as well as using a wheelchair. Had been working as a secretary in Kenya just before accident. Now married with two small children.

Alison: Road traffic accident in 1965 when 38 years old. Paralysed from waist. Employed at that time as director's assistant in television drama. Continued working in television and now a script editor in TV drama.

Alix: Paralysed at T4/5 as a result of a car accident in 1963 when she was 32 years old. Married with three young children at the time. Her husband was killed in the same accident. Has since remarried.

Amanda: Car accident in 1981 resulted in C6 lesion (complete). She was 24 at the time. Did not return to work or to her previous home, and now lives in an extension built on to her parents' house.

Amelia: Cycling accident in 1951 when 17 years old resulted in fractured spine at L1/L2. Walks with a stick. Had been working as a shorthand typist and went back to this job. Married, gave up working outside the home and then adopted a baby girl.

Amy: 'My injury was the result of an operation that went wrong.' This was in 1977 when aged 12. She is a T10 paraplegic. Could not go back to her old school and was sent to a special school. She cannot get a job. Has moved into a bungalow with her parents following her compensation award.

Andrea: Horse-riding accident in 1981 when aged 32 years. C7/8. Ran a business in London but had to give it up because three hours travelling per day was too much. Built an extension on to house where she still lives with her husband.

Angela: Car accident in 1970 when she was 20. She was paralysed from the waist down and her boyfriend was killed. At the time Angela was working as a production assistant in publishing and was living with her boyfriend. She returned to live with her parents but later bought a flat of her own. She now works in local government.

Anita: C5/6 complete as a result of a car accident in 1967 when aged 25. She had been a nurse, spent 10 years in residential care following her accident and now lives independently with her husband.

Annie: In 1978 when she was 18 years old Annie had a road accident which resulted in incomplete tetraplegia (C5) – she has arm movement and a little hand movement. She had been working as a dental nurse. After living with her mother for two years, she moved into a flat of her own. She works from home, taking telephone messages, doing bookkeeping and writing short stories.

Antonia: Tetraplegic (C4/5/6) as the result of a car accident in 1971. Unable to return to her home in Portugal, she is now in residential care in England.

Avril: Complete C5 lesion as the result of a trampolining accident in 1980. Had been a student at a polytechnic at the time but could not return. Now runs a gift shop. Lives with parents.

Barbara: C6/7 complete. Car accident on holiday in 1972 when 24 years old. A primary school teacher at the time. Now works as a school librarian.

Bernadette: Degeneration of the spinal cord (due to pernicious anaemia) left her paralysed in 1969. At the time she was married and occupied as a housewife, and she still is.

Beryl: T9/10; her injury manifested itself many years after a fall down stairs. Operated on when 66 years old in 1977 which resulted in paraplegia. Married with a grown up son. She had been a company director of a drapery and fashion business.

Beth: Accident at school in 1955 when aged 14. L1 incomplete and could walk. Moved into own flat when 22. Now wheelchair user since a knee injury. Completed university degree. Married and then divorced.

Betty: 'Run over by out of control car whilst having a family picnic.' This was in 1971 when she was aged 33 years. L3 incomplete; wheelchair user. Daughters were aged 3 and 5 and she returned to look after them.

Blanche: Fell from a window in 1961 when 31 years old. T12/L1 incomplete and can walk with sticks. Was married with three children at the time but her husband had recently left. Has done various types of work since including acting.

Brenda: Aged 52 when a horse-riding accident caused incomplete tetraplegia. Can walk short distances with sticks but mostly uses wheelchair. This happened in 1983. She was 'an active farmer's wife' working on the farm as well as running her home. Brenda's husband died soon after her accident and she now runs the farm within a partnership.

Bridget: Aged 33 in 1983 when she fell off a wall resulting in paralysis at T12. Bridget was and still is a college lecturer and a single parent.

Bronwen: 'One day my legs ached, the next they were paralysed . . . I was very frightened that the paralysis would go higher but it stopped at waist level.' This was the result of transverse myelitis in 1948 when she was 26 years old. She had been working as a children's nanny and returned to this job. When the children grew older she got a job in charge of a 'flat for rehabilitating handicapped housewives'. Now retired.

Carol: Road traffic accident when abroad in 1969. T12/L1/L2. Aged 24. Uses calipers and a wheelchair. A zoologist at the time of her accident, she returned to that area of work initially (although did not do fieldwork) but has since trained and worked as a social worker and is now taking a management course.

Caroline: In 1982 when she was 16 Caroline had an operation to move her bottom jaw forward which resulted in tetraplegia (C6). She returned to school to complete her A levels and is hoping to go to university to study law.

Catrin: Catrin was 15 years old in 1980 when a car accident resulted in paraplegia at T12. Returned to school but has not yet got a job. Is currently living with her parents.

Cecily: Injured in an accident at work in 1974 at the age of 43. After months of difficulties eventually diagnosed as having an incomplete lesion at C6. Married at the time and now divorced.

Celia: Fell from a cliff in 1964 when she was 25 years old. L1 incomplete; walks with crutches. Married at the time with a son 8½ months old. Has gained a professional qualification and is optimistic about her career prospects.

Charlotte: Road traffic accident in 1969 when she was 17. She is a complete lesion at T5. 'I still live at home with my parents and sister from choice.' Has worked as a receptionist and now works for a disability organisation.

Christine: L1/2 incomplete; walks with sticks and knee calipers. Fell off a rock at the seaside in 1958 when 21 years old; at college reading modern languages. Worked as a teacher and now is a college of education lecturer. Married when 46 years old.

Claire: Broke her back (T10) with additional damage to her right arm. She was 22 years old and was working for the Post Office. She could not return to her job but now works in a sheltered workshop. Could not return to her own home and now lives with her mother.

Claudia: Claudia was paralysed at C6 complete in 1978. She was 29 years old. Initially went into residential care but has now moved into a flat of her own.

Cora: 29 years old when she was paralysed at T6/7 as the result of a car accident.

Cynthia: T11 as the result of a car crash in 1959 when 30 years old. Had been a teacher abroad. Carried on working as a teacher for 23 years and is now retired.

Daisy: Car accident in 1952 resulted in paraplegia. She was 40 years old and a widow with two children. She had a bungalow built and still lives there with her two, grown up, sons.

Dawn: Car accident in 1972 when 23 years old. C5/6. Married with a baby girl at the time. Was in hospital for 17 months and then went into residential care. Divorced.

Deborah: Horse-riding accident in 1959 when she was almost 18. Paraplegic. Has since worked as a shorthand typist. Now lives on her own.

Denise: Fell while working on her farm in 1978. This resulted in incomplete paralysis. Uses a wheelchair but can walk short distances. 40 years old at the time and married with two sons. She returned to running her home and now does the bookwork for the farm.

Dora: Sudden paralysis when she was 13 in 1937. Walks with crutches. Was in residential care for 16 years from the age of 16. Then got married, went to work doing domestic work and later trained as a punch card operator. Did this work until retirement.

Edith: Fell down stairs in 1955 which resulted in incomplete tetraplegia. 40 years old at the time, married with two sons.

Edna: Transverse myelitis in 1983 resulted in paralysis from the waist downwards. She was 55 years old, married with four grown up children. Her life remains focused on running her home.

Eileen: Car accident in 1961 resulted in tetraplegia, C5/6. She was 14. Did not return to school. She now lives with her parents in a specially built bungalow, and is involved with various disability organisations.

Elaine: A car accident in 1969, when she was 19 years old, resulted in a lesion at C6/7/8 incomplete (wheelchair user with good use of hands). Initially moved in with parents but now lives in a flat of her own.

Elise: Paralysed at T6 complete as the result of a car accident in 1971 when 20 years old. She was an art student at the time. She has since married and has one child.

Ellen: Burst tyre caused road accident which left her paralysed at T12/L1. This was in 1970 when she was 34 years old and she was employed as a company secretary in her and her husband's painting and decorating business. The marriage ended in divorce and she now shares a home with her mother.

Elsa: Her family was ploughed into on the pavement by a speeding car. Her daughter was fatally injured, her husband severely injured but now recovered. Her other child was uninjured. This was in 1983 when Elsa was 38 and she was paralysed at T12. She had had a number of jobs working within her home, such as childminding. Returned home to care for her son and husband and has not yet taken up paid employment, although hopes to do this.

Elsbeth: Paraplegic as the result of an air crash in 1958 when aged 46. Husband killed in the same accident. Went to live with her sister. Now lives alone.

Elsie: Paralysis following a laminectomy, performed to ease the pain caused by spinal curvature. This was in the 1970s and she was in her 50s. She had been running a veterinary practice; now writes articles for journals and magazines. Married.

Emily: Car accident in 1984 when aged 43. T4/5. She was a secondary school teacher and had three children. Has not yet returned to full-time work though has done a little teaching. Still waiting to move into new house which is being adapted.

Erica: Injured her spine in the early 1960s but no major problems until 1975 when she had a lumbar fusion. In 1981 had more surgery following a car accident and again in 1982. Then remained in hospital for 18 months but developed chronic arachnoiditis caused by a series of six myelograms. 'This is a fluctuating condition and whilst the paralysis is not complete the pain factor prevents any progress toward mobility.' At that time she was a PE teacher with teenage children. Now concentrates on running her home.

Esme: Car accident in 1969 when aged 48. Married with three teenage children. T3/4. Returned home to look after her family.

Eunice: Transverse myelitis when she was 39 years old in 1964 caused paraplegia (T5/6). Married with four children (11 years to 18 months old). Returned to looking after her children and later worked part-time as a typist. Now her children are grown up she and her husband live in a bungalow and 'life is a lot easier'.

Eva: Eva was 20 when she had a car accident in 1968 which resulted in incomplete tetraplegia (C5). Went to college to do A levels and then worked as a secretary. She has since married and has two children who are both severely disabled.

Felicity: Road traffic accident in 1968. She was 30 years old and is tetraplegic (C5/6). She was working full-time and engaged to be married. She is now in residential care and has not worked since. She returned her fiancé's ring six months after the accident.

Fiona: Spinal tumour diagnosed when she was 35. Treatment with good result but recurring problems in 1980/81. Recurrence suspected and operated on with a laser. No recurrence but operation resulted in paraplegia. She is married with two teenage children and works full-time as a GP.

Fran: Car accident in 1970 at the age of 32. She is C6/7 incomplete, and a wheelchair user with the use of right hand and arm. At the time of her accident she was single with a 13-year-old daughter. Employed at the Department of Employment at the time and returned to this part-time until she left to have a family. Married, had twins, then divorced.

Frances: Car accident in 1984 when aged 21. T9/10. She was a student at the time and completed her degree. She now lives next door to her parents and is planning her future career.

Georgina: Georgina was 36 years old when a car accident resulted in tetraplegia in 1974. She was married with four sons (aged 7 to 15). As her sons grew up she and her husband moved to a smaller and more convenient house.

Geraldine: Fell off a swing in 1978 when aged 13. C5/6. Could not return to the same school and went to a special school. Cannot now pursue her ambition to be a vet. Is now married.

Gillian: Paralysed (T4) as the result of a climbing accident in 1981 when she was 23. Returned to teaching in a junior school.

Gina: Gina broke her neck (C5/6) during a dance performance in 1973 when she was 22. She was living with her boyfriend at the time and was part of a dance touring company. She broke up with her partner and eventually moved into more convenient housing. She has started a new career in costume design.

Gwen: Became paralysed from the waist down as the result of an unknown virus in 1975 when aged 17 years. Had been working as a junior clerk and living with her parents. Now married and hoping to have children.

Hannah: Tumour on spinal cord resulted in T10 lesion in 1980 when she was 32 years old. Married with two children and employed in a supermarket as a checkout operator. Returned home to look after her family. Did not go back to work.

Harriet: Car accident in 1978 resulted in T11/T12 lesion. She was 17 years old. Now works as an aviation communicator.

Hazel: Viral pneumonia caused paraplegia (T6/7) in 1971 when she was 34. She was married and had worked as a telephonist until the birth of her children, who were 2 years old and 5 months old at the time of her injury. Returned home to look after her family.

Helen: Transverse myelitis caused paraplegia (T6 complete) in 1982 when she was 27. Married with a 1-year-old daughter and eight weeks pregnant. Baby died soon after birth. Has now had another child and concentrates on looking after her two daughters.

Hilary: Hilary had a car accident in 1960 when she was 34 years old. T11. She was married with two young children at the time. She had previously worked as a health visitor but could not return to this job. Subsequently, she initially worked as a clinic clerk but is now a day centre organiser. Her husband died three years after her accident and she remarried four years after that.

Ingrid: Road accident in 1959 which resulted in a lesion at T12/L1/L2. She was 38 years old and a student nurse at the time. She had separated from her husband and was living at her parents' house with her 13-year-old daughter. Retrained as an occupational therapist and has had a successful career.

Irene: A fall in 1946 resulted in severe back pain and she had two operations in 1950. This resulted in a lot of pain, impaired sensation and a difficulty in walking. She had been working as a school matron. After living with her parents for two years she took up another school residential post and retired aged 57. She now lives with her sister and has never had a home of her own.

Isabel: T11/12 complete as the result of a suicide attempt in 1957 when she was 18. Now lives with her partner and is involved in various disability organisations.

Jackie: C4/5/6 as the result of a motorway accident in 1980 when aged 25 years old. Had left her husband shortly before and was working full-time. Now lives with her mother and is beginning to rebuild her working career.

Jacqueline: Paralysis came on over a three-week period in 1962; she is now paralysed from the waist. She was 40 at the time, married with three sons. She and her husband still live in the same house they had then which has been adapted.

Jane: Haemorrhage in 1982 when she was 38 years old caused paralysis at L2. Married with three young children. She returned to looking after her children. Jane used to be a nurse before having children and regrets that she won't now be able to return to this career.

Janet: Injured in a car accident in 1961 when 38 years old. T12. Had been working as a raincoat machinist and was a widow with two sons. Did not return to work but used a sewing machine at home. Sons are now married and Janet lives on her own.

Jean: Paralysed as the result of an accident in 1952 when she was 15. Had just started training as a glove maker. Has not done paid work since.

Jeannette: 44 years old in 1964 when a spinal tumour resulted in T12 complete lesion. Married with two teenage children and working part-time in a garage. Returned to this job working as a clerk/bookkeeper.

Jemma: 21 years old when a motor bike accident resulted in paralysis at T3/4 and a leg amputation. Her fiancé was killed. Worked at keeping house for her sister at the time. Married, had a child, then divorced. Brought up her daughter on her own.

Joyce: First hurt her back in 1964. Continual problems over the years until she became a wheelchair user in 1980. At that time married with two children. Could not go back to her part-time teaching job and now does knitting for a shop at home.

Judith: Car accident in 1970 resulted in complete lesion at T5/6. She was employed in catering and qualified in catering management. She was unable to find a job in that field but now works as a clerical officer in a hospital.

Julia: Julia had a spinal abscess in 1983 when aged 33. This caused a lesion at T1/C7. She was married with two small boys and worked part-time in a playgroup. Her husband divorced her and took the children abroad. She now looks after them in school holidays.

June: Car accident in 1980 when 57 years old. A grand-mother, and had just retired.

Karen: Car crash when 26 years old in 1975. T12/L1. At the time she was 4½ months pregnant. Child born safely at full term. Now her daughter is older, Karen is involved in a variety of disability organisations and campaigns.

Kate: C8/T1 complete as the result of a road accident in 1966 when she was 19 and at university. Completed her degree and has since lived on her own and worked in organisations concerned in one way or another with disability.

Katherine: Car accident in 1976 resulted in T10 complete lesion. She was 22 years old and had just finished college. Engaged and about to start a teaching job, she got married soon after the accident and she and her husband started their own business. They have one daughter.

Kathy: In 1979, when she had been married for a month, she had a spinal abscess which paralysed her at T10. She did not return to her job in a chemist because she had two children and hopes to have more. She childminds an 18-month-old and a 6-year-old child.

Laura: T12 complete as the result of a car accident in 1980 when 23 years old. Was working as an SRN at the time. Retrained as a social worker and now works as a hospital social worker. Now cohabiting and soon to marry.

Lauren: Sudden paralysis in 1978. Aged 34 and employed in a hospital. Living with boyfriend and children. Did not return to work. Returned to unsatisfactory housing situation and looking after her family.

Leila: Accident at stables where she worked in 1974 when she was 19. T12/L1 incomplete, she can walk. Since married and now breeds and trains dogs.

Libby: Accident at home in 1980 resulted in C4/5 incomplete. She was 17 and walks with a stick. She went to university after her accident, but having completed her degree is not sure what she wants to do. She is about to move into a flat of her own.

Lillian: Lillian had worked as a nurse and midwife. For some years she had severe back pain and was eventually operated on for a spinal fusion when she was 47 years old. This went wrong and she is now in severe pain and can hardly walk. Arachnoiditis (disease of the membrane surrounding the spinal cord) was diagnosed. She could not return to work so lost her home which went with the job (as district nurse/midwife). She moved into a small bungalow.

Linda: Car accident in 1974 when she was 33 years old. T12 complete. Linda was married with a 13-year-old daughter and worked as a college lecturer. Returned to this job but then retrained and now works as a solicitor.

Lindy: Broke her neck at C6/7 in a car accident in 1958 when she was 25. She worked as a secretary and lived with her parents. She was not able to return to work and now lives in a bungalow with her elderly mother.

Liz: Climbing accident in 1968 when 18 years old. T5/6 complete. Now married.

Lorna: 30 years old in 1974 when transverse myelitis resulted in tetraplegia (C7). Married with two sons, 5 and 6 years old. Working part-time as a secretary. Returned to look after her children; her marriage ended 10 years later.

Louise: Injured in 1985 at the age of 37 in a street accident. T5. She is married with two children aged 5 and 2 years old. At the time of filling in the questionnaire, Louise had not long been out of hospital and was still finding life very difficult, particularly as her housing situation was unsatisfactory.

Lucy: Slipped two discs as a result of lifting a patient when aged 20 in 1960. Continued working as a nurse, and then as a theatre sister, but had several breaks in her career owing to operations on her spine. Fourth operation left her with almost complete paralysis in the legs and a lot of pain. Could not continue her nursing career and is now involved in her local Dial-a-Ride as secretary of the users group. Is now married.

Lynne: Car accident in 1979 when she was 18 years old. C6 complete. Returned to (different) university to complete a degree course which she had just started. Then went to America to do postgraduate work. Now works full-time and lives on her own.

Mabel: Car accident in 1975 which resulted in T12 lesion. She was 49 years old. She had been fully occupied looking after her six children (aged from 25 to 6 years) and her father who had had a stroke. She left her husband when he started having an affair and moved into her own bungalow with the three youngest children.

Madeline: Married with three children (3, 2 and 3 months) when she had a car accident in 1964. 25 years old. Her husband was killed and she became paralysed at C7 (left side)/ T3 (right side). After 18 months was able to move into a new bungalow and look after her children.

Magda: Horse-riding accident in 1983 resulted in T5/6 lesion. She was 43 and worked as a teacher. Married with grown up children. Her husband adapted their bungalow and they still live there.

Margery: Road traffic accident in 1961. L1 incomplete. Three months pregnant at the time and two children, aged 4½ years and 18 months. Baby born safely at full term. Concentrated on looking after her family and now does voluntary work.

Margot: Motor bike accident in 1955 when she was 39 years old. T4/5. Married and very involved with helping her husband run his general practice. Returned home and eventually started working part-time. Had to give this up when husband became seriously ill. Now lives alone and looks after husband when he comes out of hospital at weekends.

Marie: A motor bike accident in 1971 when Marie was 16 years old resulted in paralysis at T5. She had just left school and worked in an office. She went to college after the accident and then returned to work in the Civil Service. Now lives in her own bungalow.

Marion: Road accident in 1983 when she was 51. Paralysed at T6 but a head injury also resulted in complete paralysis down the right side and her speech was affected. She and her husband had run a restaurant for 25 years and had three grown up children. They had to sell the restaurant and their house and moved to a bungalow.

Martha: T4 complete. Travelling in USA in 1984 when she was 26 when the van in which she was a passenger drove into the back of a stationary vehicle. Has now returned to USA and is working as a secretary/receptionist.

Mary: Road traffic accident in 1978 when she was 25 years old. T12/L1. Her daughter was just over a year old. Has since had three more children.

Mavis: Aged 34 in 1963 when a tumour was removed from her spine. Semi-ambulant for two years, wheelchair user for 10 years and now bedfast for 10 years. Had been working in a bank and teaching piano in spare time. Now, having gained accountancy qualification, does small amount of freelance accountancy work at home. Married.

Melanie: In 1969 when aged 13 Melanie had a car accident. She is now tetraplegic (C5/6). She returned to school, went on to college and then university. She now lives in a flat of her own.

Miriam: Progressive spinal arachnoiditis since she was 19 in 1959. Paraplegic since 1964. She was employed full-time for some years but then gave it up. Married.

Moira: Moira became ill with transverse myelitis in 1953 when she was 20 years old and this resulted in an incomplete T8 lesion and complete T10 lesion. She worked as a typist at the time. Subsequently she started her own small typing business, running it from home. Married in 1955.

Molly: Gradually paralysed from age of 17 as the result of a spinal tumour. Last operation in 1975 when 27 years old resulted in paraplegia. By that time married with two young children. Completed an English degree in 1982 and now does voluntary work.

Monica: Monica had a car accident in 1967 which killed her husband and broke her back at T12 complete. She was 32 years old and her children were 18 months and 3 years. Now lives in an adapted bungalow and works part-time as a clerk.

Nadia: T12 as the result of a car accident three weeks after her wedding. She was working as a university research assistant. This was in 1984, and when she filled in the questionnaire she had not long been home from hospital. Is still sorting out her housing situation and could not return to work because the building was inaccessible.

Nadine: T3/4 complete. In 1981, out walking on holiday when hit by car. Aged 38. Married, with two teenage children. Did not return to work as hospital clerk.

Naomi: Paralysed at T7 as the result of septicaemia in 1983 at the age of 35. Had been working part-time as a clerk/typist. Married. Looking for a more suitable place to live at the time of filling in the questionnaire.

Nasreen: Car accident in 1971 when she was 16 years old resulted in incomplete tetraplegia (C6/C7). Returned to school and subsequently became the first wheelchair user in Jordan to complete university.

Nicola: Road traffic accident in 1977 when she was 14 resulted in paraplegia. Now works full-time as a shorthand typist and lives on her own.

Nora: C5/6 as a result of a road accident in 1962 when she was 20 years old. Had just started teaching and did not return to this job. Did private tutoring for a while after her accident. Now married and concentrates on running her home and garden.

Norma: In 1959 Norma was nearly 17 when she was knocked down by a lorry which resulted in complete tetraplegia (C6). She was employed as a typist and had just got engaged. The relationship ended. She did not return to work and now lives with her parents.

Olivia: Motor bike accident in 1982 when she was 25 years old. T3/4 incomplete. Was working as a secretary at the time and living with her boyfriend. She returned to work and has now married.

Pamela: Car accident in 1972 when she was 23. T6 incomplete. She walks but has semi-paralysed trunk muscles, a spastic right leg and impaired bladder and bowel function and sensation. She was married and working as a teacher. She was asked to resign her teaching job but now works part-time in further education. She has had two children since her accident.

Patsy: In 1974 when Patsy was 45 years old she was run over by a car. T12 complete. At the time she was employed, and married with four children (the youngest was 10).

Paula: Paula was stabbed by her husband in 1979 when she was 29 years old. She is paraplegic. She had three children (twins aged 4 and a son aged 13). She has since emigrated, qualified and works as a teacher.

Pauline: Road traffic accident in 1981 left her with an incomplete lesion at C5/6. She was 34 years old, had three children (aged 15, 14 and 10) and was separated from her husband. She has since remarried.

Penny: Penny was 29 when she had a car accident in 1983. C6 complete. At the time of her accident she was working as an accountant. Married. Returned to work.

Phyllis: Fell in 1966 and hit her back on a kerb stone which caused paraplegia. She was 38 years old and married with a 9-year-old son. She worked in a clothing store. She could not return to work but has been involved in lots of leisure activities. Her husband died in 1970.

Polly: Hysterectomy followed by a laminectomy in 1978 left her with an incomplete lesion. Acute pain prevents her from using a wheelchair. Married at the time and employed part-time in teaching. She was 39 years old and was not able to return to work.

Rachel: Rachel was 38 years old in 1981 and living in Portugal when she fell off a wall and sustained an incomplete lesion at L1. She walks with foot splints and crutches. At the time she was employed as a secretary and had a steady boyfriend. She returned to work and also to the same home.

Ranjan: Ranjan was stabbed when she was 9 years old in 1963, and this damaged her spinal cord at C6/7. In 1982 the damage spread to C5/6. Her mother was killed in the same incident. She came to England from Pakistan for treatment and then went to boarding school in England. She now lives in a flat and teaches English as a second language.

Rebecca: Motor bike accident in 1975. T12/L1. She was 27 years old, married and working in the Civil Service. Did not return to work.

Rosalind: T11/12 complete. Traffic accident abroad in 1976 when she was 32. Returned to her job as a civil servant and is still working as such. Lives on her own.

Rosemary: Paralysed at T3 complete in 1984 when she was 27 years old. Married and working in a bank. Has returned to work but was downgraded, although she hopes to work her way up again.

Ruth: Spinal tumour when 21 years old in 1951. Before then she had cared for her father, brother and sister as her mother died when she was 13. 'My life was very hard – I just worked and looked after the house.' Her sister looked after her but eventually she moved into a bungalow on her own.

Samantha: Road traffic accident in 1976 when she was 32. 'Totally paralysed from the neck down.' Had been running her own business and was married with two sons. Was not able to carry on working but did return to look after her children with help. Her husband left 15 months after she returned home.

Sandra: Paralysis from the waist down following a cordotomy operation. This was in 1975 when she was 30 and married with three young children. Returned to look after her family.

Sarah: Fell down a flight of stairs in 1957. Gradually became paralysed over the next nine months and finally diagnosed as T10/11 complete. She was in a religious order at the time to which she could not return. Has since married.

Sheila: Injured as the result of a fall on the seafront at Blackpool. T7. This was in 1971 when she was 51 years old. Was married and working as an attendant in a home for blind people. She has a son and grandchildren.

Shirley: Shirley was 33 years old in 1981 when she had a horse-riding accident. T7. Married with three children (youngest was aged 4). Moved to a bungalow – 'Was a "housewife" previously and remain so.'

Tessa: In 1979, when she was 20 years old and a student reading mathematics, an unidentified illness left her paraplegic. Finished her degree, then worked as a consultant mathematician at a research institute. She lived with her parents until she married aged 25.

Theresa: Injured in a road traffic accident in 1975 which resulted in C7/8 incomplete lesion. She was 35 years old and was married with three sons, aged 6, 7 and 9. After difficulties with housing was able to continue looking after her children and still focuses her attention on looking after them. She and her husband divorced.

Ursula: Climbing accident when 34 years old in 1960. T7/8. Returned to original research job. Now retired.

Valerie: Valerie was 19 when she had a diving accident in 1955 which resulted in a C6 complete lesion. She was working at the GPO. She had to go into residential care but after 10 years got her own flat. She is now married.

Vicky: Paralysed at C6/7 by a virus infection in 1974 when 19 years old. A university student of music at the time, she changed her course of study to computing and is now employed in this field.

Victoria: Complete lesion at T6 in 1978 when she had just turned 18. She was living with her boyfriend and working as a stock controller in a pharmaceutical company. Split up with her boyfriend and now lives in own bungalow. Has started doing an Arts degree which she is very pleased about.

Violet: Fell downstairs at work (the Post Office) when she was 37 years old in 1968. Gradually got worse and is now a wheelchair user with acute pain. Retired on medical grounds in 1977. Married with three children. Now a widow.

Wendy: Fell downstairs at home in 1981. C5/6. Married with teenage children and employed as a welfare secretary in a school. She was 48 years old and was unable to return to her job.

Willa: Knocked over by a car when 23 years old in 1966. L5/S1. Uses calipers. Married and working in an office. Returned to her job and then gave it up to have her two children.

Yvonne: Horse-riding accident in 1984 resulted in incomplete lesion at C6/C7. Walks with sticks. She was married with a disabled teenager and two stepchildren. Worked full-time in teaching. Has returned to look after her family and also to full-time teaching.

Glossary

Abscess: a collection of pus formed anywhere in the body.

Calipers: metal supports which are strapped on to the leg and which aid walking with crutches.

Catheter: a small tube which is inserted into the urethra (through which urine passes from the bladder to its opening just in front of the vagina). It can either be left in place (attached to a drainage bag) for some days or weeks or can be inserted for a few seconds to empty the bladder.

Cervical: refers to vertebrae which support the skull and neck.

Complete paraplegia: complete loss of movement and feeling in the lower part of the body. In this context, the lower part of the body is defined as the chest down. The extent of paralysis will depend on the level of the injury (see diagram on p.00 for relationship between level of injury and groups of muscles).

Complete tetraplegia: complete loss of movement and feeling in the lower part of the body and in the hand and arm muscles which are affected by damage to the spinal cord at the different cervical levels (see diagram on p.00 for relationship between level of injury and groups of muscles).

Cyst: an abnormal sac or pouch within the body, usually filled with fluid or solid material.

Hypothermia: abnormally low body temperature, a condition which can be fatal.

Incomplete paraplegia: incomplete loss of movement and feeling in the lower part of the body.

Incomplete tetraplegia: incomplete loss of movement and feeling in all four limbs.

Incontinence: inability to control the bladder and/or bowels.

Level of lesion: level of damage to the spinal cord. This is usually described in relation to the part of the back or neck where the damage occurs. Thus, T12 means injury at the 12th thoracic vertebra; C6 means injury at the 6th cervical vertebra. Please refer to the diagram on p.00 for information about the different levels of paralysis.

Lumbar: refers to vertebrae which support the pelvis.

Non-traumatic injury: injury caused by a medical condition (such as spinal arachnoiditis) or illness (such as the virus transverse myelytis, or a tumour).

Occupational therapy: in hospitals, this assists disabled people to engage in everyday activities (for example, cooking). In the community, occupational therapists are employed as social workers or advisers to disabled people and are usually involved in sorting out housing, aids and equipment.

Paraplegia: paralysis affecting the lower part of the body, as a result of damage to the spinal cord at thoracic or lumbar (trunk) level.

Physiotherapy: physical activity which maximises the use of muscles following disability. 'Passive' physiotherapy (that is, movements of the paralysed parts of the body by a physiotherapist) may also be done to prevent contractures.

Pressure sores: a sore caused by pressure (from sitting or lying) being exerted for too long on one point, thus reducing blood supply and damaging underlying tissue.

Quadraplegia: American term for tetraplegia.

Spasms: involuntary muscle contractions in the paralysed parts of the body.

Spinal cord injury: damage to the spinal cord which is encased within the spinal column and which carries messages between the brain and the rest of the body.

Spinal injury unit: a special unit which treats people who have sustained a spinal cord injury.

Spine: 29 bones (vertebrae) which encase the spinal cord and its nerve roots.

Tetraplegia: paralysis affecting all four limbs, resulting from damage to the spinal cord at cervical (neck) level.

Thoracic: refers to vertebrae which provide anchorage for the rib cage.

Traumatic injury: injury caused by a physical force acting on the body, for example, a road traffic accident, stabbing, or a fall.

Tumour: a growth or lump caused by abnormal multiplication of body cells which may be cancerous (that is, the condition could spread to other parts of the body) or benign (that is, the condition is static).

Vertebrae: the 29 bones in the back which form the spinal column.

Resources

Organisations specifically related to spinal cord injury

SPINAL INJURIES ASSOCATION (SIA) 76 St James's Lane, London N10 3DF; tel: 01-444 2121.

The Spinal Injuries Association is a self-help group run by and for spinal cord injured people and their families and friends. As we have direct knowledge of what being paraplegic or tetraplegic means, we are able to offer our experiences as the basis of information and support services. The SIA runs a number of national services including a confidential Welfare Service and Link Scheme, an Information Service, a Care Attendant Agency, Holiday Facilities – Home and Abroad, a Personal Injury Claims Service, and produces a number of publications including *So You're Paralysed* in five languages and a quarterly newsletter full of articles and members' letters. We work closely with the spinal injury units around the country and are involved with other disability organisations, both here and abroad, for the benefit of all disabled people.

You may think, when reading this book, that our services are only provided for spinal cord injured people, but you would be wrong. The SIA is able to provide the support and information necessary, both on a practical and emotional level, to help families and friends understand the consequences of what is in most instances a sudden injury. If they are to support their relative or friend through the entire rehabilitation process and beyond, it is important that they themselves are supported.

If you want advice, information, support or just a listening ear to talk through any problems or issues, please contact us.

Northern Ireland Paraplegic Association, 26 Bridge Road, Helen's Bay, County Down; tel: 0247 653310.

Scottish Spinal Cord Injury Association, Princes House, 5 Shandwick Place, Edinburgh EH2 4RG; tel: 031-228 3827.

Welsh Council for the Disabled, Caerbragdy Industrial Estate, Bedwas Road, Caerphilly, Mid Glamorgan CF8 3SL; tel: 0222 887325.

The following list of organisations is by no means exhaustive but gives a guide to help available.

General Organisations

Information
DIAL UK, DIAL House, 117 High Street, Clay Cross, Chesterfield, Derbyshire; tel: 0246 864498.

Disabled Living Foundation, 380-384 Harrow Road, London W9 2HU; tel: 01-289 6111.

National Association of Citizens Advice Bureaux, 115-123 Pentonville Road, London N1 9LZ; tel: 01-833 2181.

RADAR (Royal Association for Disability and Rehabilitation), 25 Mortimer Street, London W1N 8AB; tel: 01-637 5400.

Group contact for women

Afro-Caribbean Self Help Voluntary Organisation, 48 East Lake Road, London SE5; tel: 01-737 3604.

Asha Asian Women's Resource Centre, c/o 27 Santley Street, London SW4; tel: 01-737 5901/274 8854.

Bristol Women with Disabilities Group, c/o Idea, William House, 101 Eden Vale Road, Westbury, Wiltshire BA13 3QF.

Disabled Women in Greenwich, c/o Ann Rae, Flat 2, 98 Woodhill, Woolwich, London SE18.

Gemma, Box 5700, London WC1N 3XX.
Gemma is a group of disabled and able-bodied lesbian women who meet on a regular basis in the London area and publish a newsletter.

Manchester Disabled Women's Group, c/o 14 Clovelly Road, Chorlton, Manchester M21 2XW.

Sisters Against Disablement (SAD), c/o Women's Reproductive Rights Information Service, 52–54 Featherstone Street, London EC1; tel: 01-251 6332.
A group of disabled women meet every month to discuss issues of feminism and disability.

Union of Physically Impaired People Against Segregation (UPIAS) Women's Group, c/o 56 Thanet Street, Clay Cross, Chesterfield, Derbyshire S45 9JT.

Winvisible (Women with visible and invisible disabilities), Kings Cross Women's Centre, 71 Tunbridge Street, London WC14 9DZ.

Women's Therapy Centre, 6 Manor Gardens, London N7; tel: 01-263 6200.
Provides individual, group therapy, and workshops on different topics – reduced prices available.

Women with Disabilities, Hackney Women's Centre, 20 Dalston Lane, London E8.

Women with Disabilities Group, c/o Anne Saunders, Equal Opportunities and Race Relations Dept., Derbyshire County Council, Council Offices, Matlock, Derbyshire D4 3AG.

Housing

Housing associations
Housing Association Liaison Office (HALO), 11A Apollo Place, London SW10; tel: 01-352 0909.
Maintains a register of people who require accommodation through housing associations in London.

Housing with care
Crossroads Care Attendant Schemes, National Office, 10 Regents Place, Rugby, Warwickshire CV21 2PN; tel: 0788 73653.
This organisation has groups all over the country who provide hours of personal care and relief help.

Grove Road Scheme, 30 Grove Road, Sutton-in-Ashfield, Nottinghamshire NG17 4LR; tel: 0623 513429.

Sheltered Housing Assistance for Disabled People (SHAD), Wandsworth Branch, Nightingale Centre, 8 Balham Hill, London SW12 9DS; tel: 01-675 6095.

Both SHAD and Grove Road provide a flat and personal assistance when needed.

Housing problems
Housing Hotline: tel: 021-359 8501/2/3 (Telephone advice service).

SHELTER, 88 Old Street, London EC1V 9HU; tel: 01-253 0202
Can provide you with details of your nearest Housing Aid Centre.

Residential accommodation
Carematch, Residential Care Consortium, 286 Camden Road, London N7 0BJ; tel: 01-609 9966
Carematch operates a computer data base which lists residential and nursing homes in the UK.

Aids, equipment and adaptations

Centre on the Environment for the Handicapped (CEH), 35 Great Smith Street, London SW1P 3BJ; tel: 01-222 7980
Provides information and advice to architects, housing planners and disabled people on adaptations to property and access to public buildings.

Disabled Living Foundation, 380–384 Harrow Road, London W9 2HU; tel: 01-289 6111.
Holds information on all aids and equipment on the market; much of which can be viewed at their office.

Possum Controls Ltd., Middlegreen Road, Langley, Slough, Berkshire SL3 6DF; tel: 0753 79234

Beds and mattresses
Egerton Hospital Equipment Ltd., Tower Hill, Horsham, West Sussex RH13 7JT; tel: 0403 53800
Produces a number of electrically operated beds.

Hoists
The Wessex Medical Equipment Co. Ltd, Unit 2, Budds Lane Industrial Estate, Romsey, Hampshire SO5 08J; tel: 0794 518246
As well as hoists, this organisation produces an electrically operated door opening device.

Toilet aids
Southern Sanitary Specialists Ltd., Cerdic House, West Portway, Andover, Hampshire SP10 3LF; tel: 0264 24131
Has a wide range of handrails for bath, toilet, shower etc.

Wheelchairs
Most manual wheelchairs will be issued by your local Artificial Limbs and Appliances Centre, but electric wheelchairs can be bought from a number of companies.

Everest and Jennings, Princewood Road, Corby, Northamptonshire NN17 2DK; tel: 0536 67661

Vessa Ltd., Papermill Lane, Alton, Hampshire GE34 2PY; tel: 0420 83294

Wheelchair seat cushions
RAYMAR, PO Box 16, Henley on Thames, Oxfordshire RG9 1AG; tel: 0491 578446

Tendercare Products Ltd., London Road, Ashington, West Sussex RH20 3JP; tel: 0903 892825

Transport

Disabled Drivers' Association, Ashwellthorpe Hall, Ashwellthorpe, Norfolk NR6 1EX; tel: 050 841 449.
Self-help association for those wanting to be mobile.

Federation of London Dial-a-Ride, St Margarets, 25 Leighton Road, London NW5 1QD; tel: 01-482 2325
Provides information on Dial-a-Ride services.

Mobility Information Service, Unit 2a, Atcham Industrial Estate, Upton Magna, Shrewsbury, SY4 4UG; tel: 0743 77489
Information on aspects of driving and assessments.

Motability, 2nd Floor, The Gatehouse, Westgate, The High, Harlow, Essex CM20 1HR: tel: 0279 635666
Provide schemes for leasing or purchasing adapted cars.

Tripscope, 63 Esmond Road, London W4 1JE; tel: 01-994 9294
Transport information for disabled people.

Access

Access Committee for England, 35 Great Smith Street, London SW1P 3BJ; tel: 01-222 7980
National focal point on access to the built environment.

Centre on the Environment for the Handicapped (CEH), 35 Great Smith Street, London SW1P 3BJ; tel 01-222 7980

Welfare rights

Child Poverty Action Group (CPAG), 1–5 Bath Street, London EC1V 9PY; tel: 01-253 3406

DHSS FREEPHONE 0800 666555

Disablement Income Group (DIG), Millmead Business Centre, Millmead Road, London N17 9QU; tel: 01-801 8013

Disability Alliance, 25 Denmark Street, London WC2 8NJ; tel: 01-240 0806

Employment

Association of Disabled Professionals, The Stables, 73 Pound Road, Banstead, Surrey SM7 2HU; tel: 07373 52366

Manpower Services Commission, Employment Division, Moorfoot, Sheffield 1 4PQ; tel: 0742 753 275
Contact usually through the Jobcentres; also provides office equipment for special needs.

Opportunities for the Disabled, 1 Bank Buildings, Princes Street, London EC2R 8EU; tel: 01-726 4963
Provides an employment service for job seekers and employers.

Further education

Most universities will have their own information on what facilities they can offer disabled students. However, Sussex, Southampton and Oxford are known to have adequate facilities.

National Bureau for Handicapped Students, 336 Brixton Road, London SW9 7AA; tel: 01-274 0565
Provides information and help in returning to education.

Open University, Office for Students with Disabilities, Walton Hall, Milton Keynes MK7 6AA.
Derek Child is currently the Adviser on the education of disabled students.

Continence management

Association of Continence Advisers, 380–384 Harrow Road, London W9 2HU; tel: 01-289 6111
Will give advice on management techniques and produces books about all aspects of continence management. Can put you in touch with a local adviser.

Many companies which supply continence equipment have their own information help lines which are usually Freephone.

Ileostomy Association of Great Britain and Ireland, Amblehurst House, Chobham, Woking, Surrey GU24 8PZ; tel: 09905 8277
Helps people return to active lives following surgery.

Urostomy Association, 'Buckland' Beaumont Park, Danbury, Essex CM3 4DE; tel: 024 541 4294
Provides help and information on stoma care.

Personal help and support

Association of Carers, First Floor, 21–23 New Road, Chatham, Kent ME4 4QJ; tel: 0634 813981

Association to Aid the Sexual and Personal Relationships of Disabled People (SPOD), 286 Camden Road, London N7 0BJ; tel: 01-607 8851
Can provide information on sexual matters as well as contact with an individual counsellor.

British Association for Counselling, 37A Sheep Street, Rugby, Warwickshire CV21 3BX; tel: 0788 78328/9
Can give you a list of professional counsellors in your local area.

Derbyshire Centre on Integrated Living (DCIL), Long Close, Cemetery Lane, Ripley, Derbyshire DE5 3HY; tel: 0773 40246
Provides general support and information, as well as a counselling service using counsellors who are themselves disabled.

DISCERN, 94 Mansfield Road, Nottingham, NG1 3HD: tel: 0602 588043
Provides a counselling service to people in the Nottingham area. Also provides training for those working with disabled people.

Lesbian Line, Box 1514, London WC1N 3XX; tel: 01-251 6911
Help and information mostly over the telephone.

Marriage Guidance Council, Herbert Gray College, Little Church, Rugby, Warwickshire CV21 3AP; tel: 0788 73241
Can provide counselling for marital problems.

Motherhood

British Agencies for Adoption and Fostering, 11 Southwark Street, London SE1 1RQ; tel: 01-407 8800
Main contact point for those wanting to adopt or foster.

British Pregnancy Advisory Service (BPAS), Austy Manor, Wootton Wawen, Solihull, West Midlands B95 6BX; tel: 05642 3225
Provides many services, including pregnancy testing, counselling, fertility investigation and artificial insemination.

Disabled Mothers Group, Disability Resources Centre, 11 Warner Road, Walthamstow, London E17.

The Family Planning Information Service, 27–35 Mortimer Street, London W1N 7RJ; tel: 01-636 7866
Provides free leaflets including booklist and advice on all family planning matters.

Maternity Alliance, 12 Britannia Street, London WC1X 9JP; tel: 01-837 1265
Pressure group and information service on maternity rights and services.

The National Childbirth Trust, 9 Queensborough Terrace, London W2 3TB; tel: 01-221 3833
Provides useful information and a national contact register for both able-bodied and disabled parents.

National Contact Register for Parents with Disabilities, 6 Forest Road, Crowthorne, Berkshire RG11 7EG; tel: 0344 773366
A register of parents with a disability.

National Council for One Parent Families, 255 Kentish Town Road, London NW5 2LX; tel: 01-267 1361
A useful contact point for single parents.

Parents for Children, 222 Camden High Street, London NW1 8QR; tel: 01-485 7526
Adoption agency for school age children and children with disabilities within 100-mile radius of London. Welcomes both single and disabled people.

Medical problems

Spinal injury units
There are, at present, nine specialist spinal units in England and Wales, two in Scotland, one in Northern Ireland and one in Eire.

The National Spinal Injuries Centre, Stoke Mandeville Hospital, Mandeville Road, Aylesbury, Bucks HP21 8AL; tel: 0296 84111

The Midland Spinal Injuries Unit, The Robert Jones and Agnes Hunt Orthopaedic Hospital, Oswestry, Shropshire SY10 7AG; tel: 0691 655311

Rookwood Spinal and Rehabilitation Unit, Rookwood Hospital, Fairwater Road, Cardiff, Wales CF5 2YN; tel: 0222 566281

The Duke of Cornwall Spinal Treatment Centre, Odstock Hospital, Salisbury, Wiltshire SP2 8BJ; tel: 0722 336262

Pinderfields General Hospital, Aberford Road, Wakefield, West Yorkshire WF1 4DG; tel: 0924 375217

Regional Spinal Injuries Centre, Promenade Hospital, Leicester Street, Southport, Merseyside PR9 0HY; tel: 0704 34411

Hexham General Hospital, Hexham, Northumberland NE46 1QJ; tel: 0434 606161

Royal National Orthopaedic Hospital, Brockley Hill, Stanmore, Middlesex; tel: 01-954 2300

Lodge Moor Hospital, Sheffield, South Yorkshire S10 4LH; tel: 0742 630222

Edenhall Hospital, Musselburgh, Midlothian, Scotland EH21 3TZ; tel: 031-665 2546

Philipshill Spinal Unit, Philipshill, Busby, Glasgow, Scotland; tel: 041-64 41144

Withers Orthopaedic Hospital, Musgrave Park Hospital, Stockman's Lane, Balmoral, Belfast BT9 7JB, Northern Ireland; tel: 0232 669501

National Medical Rehabilitation Centre, Our Lady of Lourdes Hospital, Rochestown Avenue, Dunlaoghaire, Dublin, Eire; tel: 0001 854777

Pain clinics
Most referrals to a pain clinic are through a GP or consultant. The following are well-known clinics; you can check, however, whether your local hospital has any facility of this kind.

Pain Relief Foundation, Walton General Hospital, Liverpool L9 1EA

Pain Relief Unit, The Royal Sussex Hospital, Brighton BN2 5BE

Pain Relief Unit, Abingdon Hospital, Abingdon OX14 1AG

Pain Relief Unit, The International College of Oriental Medicine, East Grinstead RH19 1TZ

Alternative Treatment
The British Hypnotherapy Association, 67 Upper Berkeley Street, London W1; tel: 01-723 4443

The British Homoeopathic Association, 27a Devonshire Street, London W1; tel: 01-935 2163

The British Acupuncture Association, 34 Alderney Street, London SW1V 4EU; tel: 01-834 1012

Foundation Offering Relief of Disability through Education, Arts and Healing (FORDEAH), PO Box 484, London NW3 4HW; tel: 01-794 9432

Consultative associations
Action for the Victims of Medical Accidents, The Hop Exchange, 24 Southwark Street, London SE1 1TY; tel: 01-403 4744
Gives advice and support to people who have suffered accidents of a medical nature and takes up individual cases.

The Patients Association, Room 33, 18 Charing Cross Road, London WC2H 0HR; tel: 01-240 0671
Gives help and advice to patients.

Back pain
Back Pain Association, 31–33 Park Road, Teddington, Middlesex TW11 0AB; tel: 01-977 5474
Has an information service for people sufffering from back complaints.

Aging

Centre on Policy for Aging, 25–31 Ironmonger Row, London EC1V 3QP; tel: 01-253 1787
Is an independent body set up to do research on aging. Has a useful library which can be used by appointment. Not a specialist organisation in disability.

Leisure

British Sports Association for the Disabled, Hayward House, Barnard Crescent, Aylesbury, Bucks HP21 9PP; tel: 0296 27889
Provides information on all sports, clubs and games available to disabled people.

Friends by Post, 6 Bollin Court, Maclesfield Road, Wilmslow, Cheshire SK9 2AP
Offers conversation by correspondence to try to combat loneliness.

International Correspondence Service, PO Box 10, Matlock, Derby.
Free pen-friendship service for disabled people.

Physically Handicapped and Able-Bodied Club (PHAB), Tavistock House North, Tavistock Square, London WC1H 9HX; tel: 01-388 1963
Clubs and holidays are organised to bring disabled and able-bodied people together.

The Outsiders Club, PO Box 4ZB, London W1A 4ZB; tel: 01-741 3332
This is a club designed to help both disabled and able-bodied people meet for friendship and partnership.

SHAPE, 1 Thorpe Close, London W10 5XL; tel: 01-960 9245
Arts workshops and projects with, by and for disabled people. Runs a ticket scheme for access to London's arts venues; tel: 01-960 9249.

Sportsline: tel: 01-222 8000
Advises on sports/activities for women and facilities for disabled women.

Holidays and travel

RADAR (Royal Association for Disability and Rehabilitation), 25 Mortimer Street, London W1N 8AB; tel: 01-637 5400
RADAR publishes holiday and motoring guides for the disabled traveller.

Holiday Care Service, 2 Old Bank Chambers, Station Road, Horley, Surrey RH6 9NW; tel: 0293 774 535
Specialises in organising holidays with a helper for disabled people.

Threshold Travel, 2 Whitworth Street West, Manchester M1 5WX; tel: 061-236 9763
Travel agent specialising in holidays for disabled people.

Winged Fellowship Trust, Angel House, Pentonville Road, London N1 9XD; tel: 01-833 2594
Provides holidays for severely disabled people.

Bibliography

Brown, Susan, Connors, Debra and Stern, Nanci (eds), *With the Power of Each Breath – A Disabled Woman's Anthology*, Cleis Press, PO Box 14684, San Francisco, CA 94114, 1985.
'A work of resistance against institutionalised silence.' A collection of stories abour growing up, speaking out, anger, sexism, oppression, self-image, friendship, love and motherhood.

Campling, Jo (ed), *Images of Ourselves – Women with Disabilities Talking*, Routledge & Kegan Paul, 1981.
Women with a range of disabilities talk about their lives.

Cornwell, M., *Early Years*, Disabled Living Foundation, 1975.
Practical ideas about looking after children if you're disabled.

Deegan, Mary Jo and Brooks, Nancy A (eds), *Women and Disability, the Double Handicap*, Transaction Books, Rutgers University, New Brunswick, New Jersey 08903, 1985.
Articles examining the negative stereotyping of disabled women, sexuality, assertiveness, motherhood, etc.

Duffy, Yvonne, *All Things are Possible*, A.J. Garvin & Associates, PO Box 7525, Ann Arbor, MI 48107, 1983.
Written by a disabled woman, this book is about sexuality and is based on interviews with women with a range of disabilities.

Fallon, Bernadette, *So You're Paralysed*, 2nd edition, Spinal Injuries Association, 1987.
The definitive introductory guide for the newly paralysed person, her family and friends. Available from the SIA.

Ferguson Matthews, Gwyneth, *Voices From the Shadows*, The Women's Press, 16 Baldwin Street, Toronto, Ontario, Canada, 1983.
Based on interviews with women with a range of disabilities and covering all aspects of their lives.

Grundy, D, Russell, J and Swain, A, *ABC of Spinal Cord Injury*, British Medical Journal, 1986.

Principally written for the medical and allied professions, this is a concise and comprehensive guide to the management of spinal cord injury from the point of injury to final discharge from hospital.

Hannaford, Susan, *Living Outside Inside, A Disabled Woman's Experience*, Canterbury Press, Box 2151C, Berkeley, CA 94702, 1985.

A collection of writings on disability from a socialist feminist perspective.

McCarthy, B, *Disabled Eve*, Disabled Living Foundation, 1981.

A guide to coping with menstruation for disabled women.

Maddox, Sam, *Spinal Network – The Total Resource for the Wheelchair Community*, Spinal Network, PO Box 4162, Boulder, CO 80306, 1987.

A US reference work containing comprehensive information on a wide range of aspects of spinal cord injury with a mixture of factual and personal detail.

Rogers, Michael, *Paraplegia*, 2nd edition, Faber & Faber, 1986.

A handbook of practical care and advice. Topics covered include prevention and care of pressure sores, bladder and bowel management, sexuality, adjusting to community life after hospital discharge, holidays, travel and other topics. The author is spinal cord injured.

Saxton, Marsha and Howe, Florence (eds), *With Wings, An Anthology of Literature By and About Women with Disabilities*, Virago, 1988.

First published in the USA this book has an introduction by Merry Cross.

Shearer, Ann, *Living Independently*, CEH and Kings Fund, 1982.

Details accounts of the practicalities of independent living for nine severely disabled people, including photographs and plans of housing as well as information about personal care provision. It is available from the Centre on Environment for the Handicapped, 126 Albert Street, London NW1 7NF.

Spinal Injuries Association, *Spinal Cord Injuries – Guidance for General Practitioners and District Nurses*, SIA.

This manual, available from the SIA, provides general practitioners, district nurses and carers with clear information on the needs of paralysed people in the community. It explains symptoms unique to paraplegia and tetraplegia and provides details of treatment. It also contains a list of where to obtain equipment.

Spinal Injuries Association, *Nursing Management in the General Hospital – The First 48 Hours Following Injury*, SIA.
This manual, available from the SIA, provides clear guidance to general nursing staff who may be inexperienced in the nursing of people with suspected spinal cord injuries.

Sutherland, Allan T, *Disabled We Stand*, Souvenir Press, 1981.
A political analysis of disablity issues using interviews with a group of people with a range of disabilities.

Trieschmann, Roberta, *Spinal Cord Injuries – Psychological, Social and Vocational Adjustment*, Pergamon Press, 1980.
Written mainly for professionals but of great interest to spinal cord injured people. Covers the consequences of injury and the psychological and social factors associated with disablity. The book is a landmark in this field as it explodes a number of myths and is particular important in that it draws on the experiences of spinal cord injured people themselves.